KT-511-693

The Ethnic Health Handbook

A Factfile for Health Care Professionals

Edited by

Ghada Karmi
MB, PhD, MRCP, FFPHM
Specialist in Public Health
Former Head of the Regional Health
and Ethnicity Programme, London

UNIVERSITY OF CENTRAL
LANCASHIRE LIBRARY
BLACKPOOL SITE

Blackwell
Science

BLACKPOOL, FYLDE AND WYRE
NHS LIBRARY

TV11292

© 1996 by
Blackwell Science Ltd
Editorial Offices:
Osney Mead, Oxford OX2 0EL
25 John Street, London WC1N 2BL
23 Ainslie Place, Edinburgh EH3 6AJ
238 Main Street, Cambridge,
  Massachusetts 02142, USA
54 University Street, Carlton,
  Victoria 3053, Australia

Other Editorial Offices:
Arnette Blackwell SA
  1, rue de Lille, 75007 Paris
  France

Blackwell Wissenschafts-Verlag GmbH
  Kurfürstendamm 57
  10707 Berlin, Germany

  Feldgasse 13, A-1238 Wien
  Austria

All rights reserved. No part of this publication
may be reproduced, stored in a retrieval
system, or transmitted, in any form or by any
means, electronic, mechanical, photocopying,
recording or otherwise, except as permitted by
the UK Copyright, Designs and Patents Act
1988, without the prior permission of the
publisher.

First published 1996

Set in 10/12pt Souvenir
by DP Photosetting, Aylesbury, Bucks
Printed and bound in Great Britain
by Hartnolls Ltd., Bodmin, Cornwall

DISTRIBUTORS

Marston Book Services Ltd
PO Box 87
Oxford OX2 0DT
(*Orders:* Tel: 01865 791155
         Fax: 01865 791927
         Telex: 837515)

North America
  Blackwell Science, Inc.
  238 Main Street
  Cambridge, MA 02142
  (*Orders:* Tel: 800 215-1000
           617 876-7000
           Fax: 617 492-5263)

Australia
  Blackwell Science Pty Ltd
  54 University Street
  Carlton, Victoria 3053
  (*Orders:* Tel: 03 347-0300
           Fax: 03 349-3016)

A catalogue record for this book is available
from the British Library

ISBN 0–632–04042–4

Library of Congress
Cataloging-in-Publication Data

The ethnic health handbook: a factfile for
  health care professionals/edited by
  Ghada Karmi.
      p.   cm.
    Includes bibliographical references and
index.
    ISBN 0–632–04042–4 (alk. paper)
    1. Transcultural medical care—Great
Britain–Handbooks, manuals, etc.
2. Minorities—Medical care—Great Britain
—Handbooks, manuals, etc.
I. Karmi, Ghada.
RA418.5.T73E84   1995
362.1'08'693—dc20   95-38399
                                  CIP

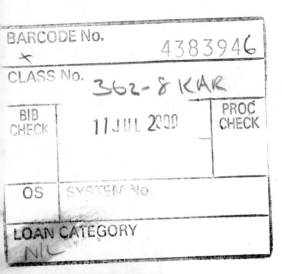

BARCODE No.
✗   4383946

CLASS No. 362-8 KAR

BIB
CHECK   11 JUL 2000   PROC
                             CHECK

OS   SYSTEM No.

LOAN CATEGORY
  NC

Contents

Preface

This book derives from an earlier publication, *The Ethnic Health Factfile*, which was first published in 1992 by the Health and Ethnicity Programme of the NW/NE Thames Regional Health Authorities. The earlier book was presented in ring-binder form and was meant to act as a personal factfile for users who could add their own comments and observations to the text. It was an instant success and sold out in two printings. Because of its evident usefulness to practitioners, the decision was taken to re-issue the book, but this time to expand and update the contents in line with the feedback received from readers of the first edition. Hence, the present book.

The main purpose of *The Handbook* is to provide rapidly assimilable information to health care professionals who deal with ethnic minority patients. One of the more regrettable aspects of health care for ethnic minorities in Britain has long been the widespread ignorance of health professionals at all levels about non-British cultures and customs. This originates from an almost total lack of training in multi-cultural health care at medical and nursing schools which hardly improves at the post-graduate stage. While many ethnic minority customs have no bearing on health, a few of them are crucially important for the provision of culturally appropriate and sensitive health care. Furthermore, patterns of disease are known to differ between ethnic groups, and this needs to be recognised for diagnosis and treatment to be effective. It is for these reasons that *The Handbook* was compiled.

The book is a quick and handy guide, summarising for each ethnic group the major facts that are relevant to health care. Each entry is set out systematically, using similar sub-headings throughout for ease of reference. The material is presented in abbreviated form, so as to enable busy practitioners to glean the information they need, virtually at a glance. In addition to the ethnic group entries, a number of sections on subjects of general relevance have been compiled. These include a demographic profile of the ethnic minority population in today's Britain, as derived from the 1991 census; a summary of refugee health issues, which are likely to gain in importance as the number of refugees and asylum seekers increases world-wide; and last, but not least, a special entry on ethnic monitoring. This procedure became mandatory for all in-patients in England on 1 April 1995, at a time when many of those who were to be engaged in ethnic monitoring were unfamiliar and unpractised in the technique. The ethnic monitoring section in the present book summarises the main aspects of this important procedure.

The ethnic groups which have been included were selected firstly because of their size (approximately more than 5000), and secondly, because factors connected with their ethnicity have a relevance to health care. Even so, it is possible that some groups could have been missed. One group in particular whose omission from the book may arouse debate is the Irish community. The Irish have not been traditionally viewed as 'ethnic' because they are white and speak English as their mother tongue (excepting a small number who use Gaelic). Recently, however, some Irish people have begun to question this assumption. They argue that the Irish face the same problems of prejudice, poor housing and social hardship as many other migrants, and have specific health problems. Irish people in Britain have the highest psychiatric admission rates and the highest rates for alcohol dependence of any group. On all these grounds, they should qualify for inclusion as an ethnic minority. While the facts are not in dispute, we have nevertheless taken the view in this book that the definition of an 'ethnic' minority must have a cut-off point, otherwise, using the same logic, we could have included the Welsh and the Scottish also as 'ethnic minorities'.

The Handbook does not claim to be fully comprehensive. It is merely intended to act as a quick reference for the most important facts relating to each group. Consultation was sought widely from ethnic community leaders, where possible, and from health workers dealing with black and ethnic minorities. While the responses were mostly positive, the criticism was made that *The Handbook* might encourage the stereotyping of ethnic minorities. It is likely that this danger will be inherent in any synopsis, and we have tried to avoid the use of descriptions which could give that impression. We can only hope that we have succeeded. If not, then we would wish to apologise in advance for any offence to any community member which might be inadvertently caused by the information in this book.

Ghada Karmi

Acknowledgements

I wish to acknowledge with gratitude the excellent work of my research assistant, Malcolm Hashemi, who is responsible for a major share of the research and writing of this book.

Special thanks are due also to the following people whose expert knowledge of their communities provided us with valuable insights and made the compilation of *The Handbook* in its present form possible: Tekle Berhe, Eritrean Community in the UK; Esme Daniels, Board of Deputies of British Jews; Dr Ganesh Dutt, Bethnal Green Health Centre; Dympna Edwards, North Thames Regional Health Authority; Dr Girma Ejere, Ethiopian Community in Britain; Dr Gene Feder, St Bartholomew's Hospital Medical College; Myra Garrett, Mohamud Ahmad, Shamsu Alam, Rahima Hussein and Jahanara Loqueman, Tower Hamlets Health Strategy Group; Gopal Ghandi, Indian Embassy; Mathur Krishnamurthi, Institute of Indian Culture; Dr Pui Ling Li, London Chinese Health Resource Centre; Ron Maddox, Buddhist Society; Evan Millner and Jess Clare, Jewish Care; Dr Nadia, Sudanese Community Information Centre; Misak Ohanian, Centre for Armenian Information and Advice (CAIA); Jenik Parijanian, Iranian Community Centre; Professor Harminder Singh, Sikh Divine Fellowship; Jessica Yudilevich, Kate Allen and Julia Purcell, Refugee Council.

I would also like to thank all the representatives of organisations who provided us with updated facts and figures about the ethnic and religious groups in this country and who helped us to find suitable contacts, addresses and sources of information.

Ghada Karmi

Glossary of Religious Terms

Buddhism

Dana   generosity or unselfishness.
Karma   the sum of a person's good or bad actions in a previous life that determines his/her present and future fate.
Mahayana   populist non-orthodox branch of Buddhism prevalent in China and Japan.
Nirvana   state of perfect contentment attained when the soul is freed from suffering caused by selfish desires.
Parinirvana   complete passing away of the Buddha.
Silas   the five rules of conduct: do not kill; do not steal; be honest; abstain from intoxicating substances; and refrain from improper sexual conduct.
Therevada   orthodox school of Buddhism prevalent in India, Sri Lanka and South East Asia.
Ullumbana   Buddhist New Year and feast of all souls.
Wesak   celebration of the birth of Buddha and his entry into eternal nirvana.

Hinduism

Arti   offerings to the gods.
Bhagavaid Gita   the most important holy script for Hindus.
Bindi   red spots worn by women on their foreheads to indicate they are married.
Brahmin   the highest caste in the Hindu religion.
Caste   social category inherited at birth.
Diwali   festival of light held in October.
Ishta devata   a family's chosen deity (somewhat akin to a patron saint).
Janeu   sacred thread worn over the right shoulder and around the body.
Janmastami   birthday of Krishna.
Karma   the sum of a person's good or bad actions in a previous life that determines his/her present and future fate.
Krishna   one of the most important Hindu gods.
Mahashivaratri   celebration of the birth of Lord Shiva, held in February or March.

Mangal sutra   gold brooch worn by married women.
Om   mystical symbol of the Supreme Spirit.
Puja   family prayer room.
Pujani   Hindu priest.
Ram Navami   celebration of the birth of Lord Ram, who is the incarnation of the god Vishnu.
Sindur   dye used by newly wedded women to colour the parting of their hair.

Islam

Allah   God.
Bayram   feast marking the beginning of the month of pilgrimage to Mecca (Id al-Adha in Arabic).
Burka   headscarf used by Bangladeshi women.
Chador   Persian/Urdu for large veil or tunic worn by women for modesty (corresponds to *hijab*).
Faqih or *Fqih*   traditional faith healer.
Gibla   *see* qibla.
Hajj   pilgrimage to the holy city of Mecca that must be undertaken at least once in a lifetime, lasting about two weeks.
Halal   meat slaughtered in the ritual manner, by cutting the animal's jugular vein to drain out the blood.
Haram   forbidden by Islam.
Hijab   religious dress for women (usually a cloak or long coat and head-scarf), corresponds to *chador* worn in Iran.
Id al-Adha   (Bayram in Urdu and Turkish) feast marking the start of the holy month of pilgrimage (hajj).
Id al-Fitr   feast marking the end of the fasting month of Ramadan.
Khitan or *Khatna*   circumcision (male).
Mawlid al-Nabi   birthday of the Prophet Mohammad.
Muslim   follower of Islam and member of the Umma.
Namaaz   prayer.
Qibla   direction of Mecca, and of prayer.
Qur'an (Koran or Coran)   holy book of Muslims containing the teachings of the Prophet Mohammad, as revealed to him by Allah.
Ramadan   lunar month during which Muslims abstain from eating, smoking, drinking and sexual activity from dawn to dusk.
Rouzeh or *Rowza*   Persian and Urdu terms for fasting.
Umma   the entire community of Muslim believers – those who have embraced the faith.

Judaism

Ashkenazi   Jews originating from Eastern and Central Europe.
Bar Mitzvah   ceremony marking a young boy's entry to adulthood.
Bat Mitzvah   ceremony marking a girl's attainment of womanhood (recently adopted by Progressive Jews).
Chanukah   festival of candles held in mid-December.
Haredim   the Orthodox religious community.
Hassidim   East European (Ashkenazi) branch of the Orthodox community who tend to adopt a special rabbi as their leader.
Kappel   small skullcap worn by observant Jewish men.
Kosher   permitted food i.e. approved by a Rabbi, and, in the case of meat, ritually slaughtered by cutting the jugular vein to allow the blood to drain out.
Lubavitch   ultra-Orthodox sect of the Hassidim.
Misnagdim   non-Hassidic Haredim, who do not follow a particular leader.
Mohel   person qualified to perform circumcisions.
Payot   distinctive locks of hair worn by Hassidic Jews.
Pesach   Passover – eight-day festival celebrating the exodus of Jews from Egypt.
Purim   feast celebrating the deliverance of the Jews from Persia.
Rabbi   Jewish priest.
Rosh Hashanah   Jewish New Year, in September/October.
Scheitel   scarf or wig worn by Orthodox Jewish women to cover their hair in public.
Sephardi   Jews originating from Spain, North Africa and the Middle East.
Shabbat   Sabbath or Saturday – the weekly day of rest.
Shavuot   harvest festival and celebration of the revelation of the Torah on Mount Sinai (Pentecost).
Shivah   period of mourning following death.
Sukkot   autumn harvest festival commemorating the forty years of Jewish exile from Egypt (Tabernacles).
Tallit katan   fringed undergarment worn by Orthodox Jewish men.
Talmud   book of religious law, as interpreted by religious scholars from the Torah.
Tisha B'av   one day fast in August to commemorate the destruction of the Temple.
Torah   Jewish holy book and first of the five books of the Bible (Old Testament).
Treifa   prohibited food.
Yom ha-Din   Judgement Day.
Yom Kippur   Day of Atonement, marking the end of the ten days of judgement.

Sikhism

Diwali   festival of light (the triumph of good over evil) held in October.
Dupatta   religious scarf.
Gurdwara   temple.
Gurpurb   commemorative occasion or feast day.
Hola   three-day pageant commemorating Sikh military victories, held in the early spring.
Jhatka or *chakar*   meat from animals which have been ritually slaughtered with one stroke.

Five Ks

Kaccha   symbolic undershorts worn by all Sikh men.
Kangha   comb worn by Sikh men in their hair.
Kara   steel bangle talisman.
Kesh   uncut hair.
Kirpan   symbolic dagger carried by Sikh men.

Kameez or *kurta*   traditional long shirt or blouse.
Karma   the sum of a person's good or bad actions in a previous life that determines his/her present and future fate.
Kaur   title given to all Sikh women, meaning 'prince'. (The term 'prince' was originally bestowed on women in an attempt to bring their status closer to that of men. However, Kaur is generally translated as 'princess' to avoid confusion.)
Khalsa   religious order into which all Sikhs are baptised on the thirteenth day after birth.
Mela   festival.
Pagri   turban worn by most Sikh men.
Patka   inner turban used to wrap the hair.
Shalwar kameez   loose trousers and long blouse worn by Sikh women.
Singh   title given to all Sikh men, meaning 'lion'.
Vaid or *Vayid*   traditional healer.
Vaisakhi   Sikh New Year, celebrated in April.

Part 1

The Ethnic Minority Population of Great Britain

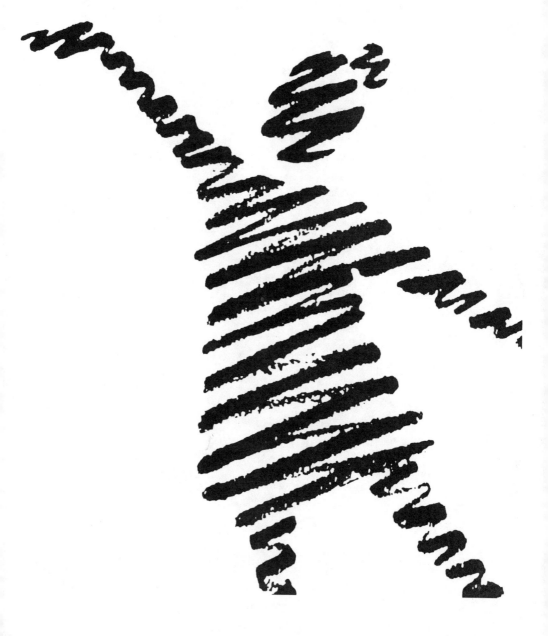

Regional Distribution of the Population

The 1991 Census of Population included for the first time a question on the ethnic group of respondents. This made it possible for the size and type of ethnic minority communities to be assessed at local authority, ward and enumeration level, and hence in health districts and family health service authorities (FHSAs). Prior to this census, the main source of statistical information on the ethnic minority population of Great Britain had been the Labour Force Survey, and this remains the only source between censuses. The Labour Force Survey samples 250 000 people every year (from 1992) and records their ethnic group according to ten categories which are similar to, but not identical with, the nine ethnic group categories in the census.

The great advantage of the ethnic population information derived from the 1991 census is that it helped to remove the previous reliance on country of birth as a proxy for ethnicity. This is no longer a satisfactory measure of ethnicity since there are increasing numbers of second generation migrants, that is people born here from ethnic parents. Furthermore, country of birth figures do not distinguish between Indian-born British expatriates and those people originally from India who were born in East Africa. Nevertheless, retaining this statistic in the last census in addition to the new ethnicity category means that it is possible to arrive at a population figure for second generation migrants. Unfortunately, the census is not able to provide data on the size of the refugee population, since this is subsumed under the ethnicity category. Estimates for this population can be derived from Home Office records of numbers of asylum applications received per year. Thus, in 1994, the total number of applications from refugees was 32 830 (source: Home Office, personal communication).

The 1991 census found that the total ethnic minority population in England and Wales was 5.9 per cent of the population (Fig. 1). For Britain as a whole, the figure falls to 5.5 per cent. The ethnic minority population is not evenly distributed, but is clustered in different localities which tend to be urban. The census found that less than one per cent of ethnic minorities lived in rural areas. England has a 6.2 per cent ethnic minority population, while in Scotland ethnic minorities constitute only 1.3 per cent of people. Over half of the ethnic minority population lives in the South East, where it forms 9.9 per cent of the total. The major concentration of ethnic minorities is to be found in

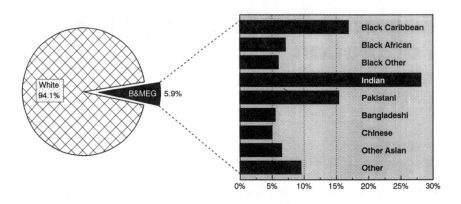

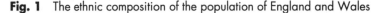

Fig. 1 The ethnic composition of the population of England and Wales

B&MEG = Black and minority ethnic groups
Source: 1991 Census, Small Area Statistics
Reproduced with the permission of the Controller of Her Majesty's Stationery Office.
© Crown Copyright

Greater London, which has 20.2 per cent of the total. Other major concentrations are to be found in the West Midlands with 8.2 per cent and Yorkshire and Humberside with 4.4 per cent (see Table 1).

Within these geographical areas, there are significant differences between ethnic group concentrations. Of Britain's 20 districts and boroughs with the highest proportions of ethnic groups, 16 are in London. The other four are Leicester, Slough, Birmingham and Luton. Brent and Newham lead with ethnic minority concentrations of 44.8 per cent and 42.3 per cent respectively, but four other London boroughs – Tower Hamlets, Hackney, Ealing and Lambeth – have over 30 per cent ethnic minority populations. The largest out-of-London ethnic minority population is to be found in Leicester, where it constitutes 28.5 per cent of the total.

Among Britain's ethnic minority population, the largest single group is Indian (Fig. 1), constituting 1.5 per cent of the population or 28 per cent of the ethnic minority population as a whole. The second largest group is the Black Caribbean group, making 16.9 per cent of the total ethnic population. But when this group is combined with the 'Black African' and 'Black Other' categories (as defined in the census), it forms 1.8 per cent of Britain's population and 30 per cent of the ethnic minority population (see Table 2).

The pattern of ethnic group clustering within districts and boroughs is interesting. Tower Hamlets has the largest concentration of Bangladeshis in the country (23 per cent), while Pakistanis form the dominant group in Birmingham, Slough, Waltham Forest and Luton. The proportion of Indian people is highest in Leicester at 22.3 per cent. But it is also high in the London boroughs of Brent, Ealing, Hounslow and Harrow at between 16 and

Table 1 Great Britain's population by ethnic group and region (1991)

| | Thousands and percentages | | | | | | |
	Black[1]	IPB[2]	Other MEGs[3]	All MEGs	White	Total pop.	MEGs as a % of total pop.
England	875	1 431	605	2 911	44 144	47 055	6.2
North	5	21	13	39	2 988	3 027	1.3
Yorkshire and Humberside	37	144	33	214	4 623	4 837	4.4
East Midlands	39	120	29	188	3 765	3 953	4.8
East Anglia	14	14	15	43	1 984	2 027	2.1
South East	610	691	395	1 695	15 513	17 208	9.9
Greater London	*535*	*521*	*290*	*1 346*	*5 334*	*6 680*	*20.2*
Rest of South East	*75*	*170*	*104*	*349*	*10 179*	*10 529*	*3.3*
South West	22	17	24	63	4 547	4 609	1.4
West Midlands	102	277	45	424	4 726	5 150	8.2
North West	47	147	50	245	5 999	6 244	3.9
Wales	9	16	16	42	2 794	2 835	1.5
Scotland	6	32	24	63	4 936	4 999	1.3
Great Britain	891	1 480	645	3 015	51 874	54 889	5.5

[1] Black Caribbean, Black African and Black other
[2] Indian, Pakistani and Bangladeshi
[3] Minority Ethnic Groups
B&MEG = Black and minority ethnic groups
Source: 1991 Census, Small Area Statistics
Reproduced with the permission of the Controller of Her Majesty's Stationery Office. © Crown Copyright

Table 2 The ethnic composition of the population of England and Wales

Ethnic group	Numbers (000s)	Per cent
White	46 937	94.1
Black Caribbean	499	1.0
Black African	205	0.4
Black other	176	0.4
Indian	830	1.7
Pakistani	455	0.9
Bangladeshi	159	0.3
Chinese	147	0.3
Other Asian	193	0.4
Other	281	0.6
B&MEG	2 945	5.9
England and Wales	49 890	100.0

B&MEG = Black and minority ethnic groups
Source: 1991 Census, Small Area Statistics
Reproduced with the permission of the Controller of Her Majesty's Stationery Office.
© Crown Copyright

17 per cent. The majority of Black Caribbean and Black African people live in London, by contrast to the Pakistani community which lives mainly in West Yorkshire and the West Midlands. About a third of the Indian minority lives in Outer London with a second smaller concentration in the West Midlands. Just over a third of the Chinese minority lives in London, where they are remarkably evenly distributed between boroughs. There is also a sizeable concentration of Chinese in north-west England.

Unfortunately, because the census has simplified ethnic categories by merging them into single groups (e.g. Punjabis, Gujaratis and Tamils are covered by the term 'Indian'), population figures for the majority of ethnic minority groups covered in this book are unavailable.

Finally, one interesting feature of the ethnic minority population is its age structure. In general, ethnic minority groups tend to have a younger age distribution than the population as a whole. Three in five people from ethnic groups are under the age of 30, compared with two in five in the population as a whole. In the Bangladeshi, Pakistani and 'Black Other' groups, about half are under the age of 16. As an average of all ethnic minority groups, a third are under 16, whereas in whites this figure is just under a fifth.

Further reading

Haskey, J. (1991) The ethnic minority populations resident in private households – estimates by county and metropolitan district of England and Wales. *Population Trends*, **63**, 22–35.

Ethnic Monitoring

Ethnic monitoring has become a subject of increasing importance in the Health Service since 1990. Interest has traditionally focused on the monitoring of employment practices, but the concept of monitoring ethnicity in the use of health services is now prominent. This is in large measure due to the priority placed on the subject by the Department of Health: ethnic monitoring of in-patients in England is now a mandatory requirement, as from 1 April 1995.

Definition

Ethnic monitoring is the process of recording ethnic origin, analysing and interpreting the results, and using the information to modify and improve practice. It is often taken to mean ethnic recording only, without any impli-cation of further action. But it is in fact a circular process, where the data collected is fed back and is used to inform subsequent practice.

Aims

The aims of ethnic monitoring are to:

- assess the use of services by ethnic groups;
- identify the health needs of ethnic groups, by using proxy information derived from service use;
- identify gaps in health service provision to ethnic groups;
- measure the outcome of service changes created in response to identified deficiencies.

Stages

Data collection

This involves: designating and training the health staff who will collect the ethnic group data; deciding on the most appropriate ethnic origin classifica-tion; and amending computer software to accept ethnic origin codes.

The classification systems should always be based on the 1991 census ethnic categories, but may be augmented by additional categories to reflect local populations.

Storage and analysis of data

Access to patients' case notes and computer records must be subject to the rules of confidentiality. Only anonymised and aggregated information can be used. After collection, the data is interpreted and analysed for answers it can provide to questions of service use, health status, and shortcomings of health service provision.

Use of data

It is important for the results of ethnic monitoring to be fed into the process of health-needs assessment and service planning. It does not in itself provide the solutions, but is a tool to identify problems and direct further action and research.

Monitoring the changes

Following a change in the delivery of services, as a result of the information provided by ethnic monitoring, the process itself monitors the effects of these changes, if any.

Practical issues

Ethnic monitoring in service provision is a new procedure for the Health Service. Little has been written on the method to be employed, and there are some practical issues of importance for those who must carry it out. The major points are summarised below.

Who should collect the information? Staff who normally collect patients' registration details should do this, as part of the same process. They should be trained appropriately.

How should the information be collected? All new patients presenting to hospital are asked to self-classify their ethnicity on special forms. The information is then transferred as part of the usual medical records procedures.

What training should staff receive? This should include an explanation of: the reasons for monitoring; the method of collection; the ethnic classification to be used; and confidentiality procedures. It should also raise staff awareness of the cultures and health needs of ethnic minorities.

What resource implications are there? Specific expense will be incurred through staff training and the integration of a new data collection item into routine recording systems.

Who is responsible for ethnic monitoring? This is probably the most important issue of all. For the process to be worthwhile, it is imperative that a designated officer with the appropriate seniority should be in charge. This officer will be responsible for the practical management of the whole operation and accountable to senior staff for its results.

Advantages

If properly implemented, ethnic monitoring can provide valuable information on the epidemiology of disease in ethnic groups. It can also reveal inequalities of access. The information can be used to make changes which should go towards improving the service and ensuring that it is sensitive, equitable and appropriate.

Reservations

If the process is used merely to record ethnicity, without a consequent change in health practice, then it may arouse the suspicion that it collects 'race data' for clandestine use. Raising patients' expectations that ethnic monitoring will create a better service for them with consultation and feedback, if not fulfilled, will be worse than if it had never been introduced in the first place.

Further reading

Karmi, G. & Horton, C. (1992) *Guidelines for the Implementation of Ethnic Monitoring*. The Health and Ethnicity Programme. NE and NW Thames Regional Health Authorities, London.
National Health Service Executive (1994) *Collecting Ethnic Group Data for Admitted Patient Care*. Department of Health, London.

Refugees and Asylum Seekers

According to the 1951 UN Convention on the Status of Refugees, a refugee is defined as:

'... a person who, owing to a well-founded fear of being persecuted for reasons of race, religion, nationality, membership of a particular social group or political opinion, is outside the country of nationality and is unable or, owing to such fear, unwilling to return to it'.

People requesting refugee status are normally referred to as asylum seekers. When requests are approved, applicants are either granted 'exceptional' or, if circumstances in the country of origin are deemed long-term, 'indefinite' leave to remain and/or refugee status. Once this has been granted, refugees may be joined by their immediate family members.

The major refugee groups in Britain are: Eritreans, Ethiopians, Ghanaians, Iranians, Kurds, Nigerians, Palestinians, Somalis, Sri Lankans (mainly Tamils), Ugandans and Vietnamese. The most recent refugee groups to arrive are from Angola, Zaire, Iraq, Somalia, Sierra Leone and the former Yugoslavia, notably Bosnia. Of the 1050 asylum seekers from the former Yugoslavia between 1 January and 30 September 1994, 905 have been granted 'exceptional leave to remain' which amounts to temporary refugee status. Only 15 were granted 'indefinite' leave to remain. About 90 per cent of refugees settle in Greater London. Not every refugee group has been included in the text, and the aim of this section is mainly to draw attention to the aspects of refugees that are relevant to health care.

Refugee communities share a number of problems. These include language difficulties and culture-shock, feelings of isolation, vulnerability and stress. Refugees have all faced persecution in one form or another, and suffer varying degrees of physical and psychological trauma; some may also have been tortured. In addition, refugees often feel insecure because of separation from their families and their uncertain legal status. This insecurity has been aggravated by the 1993 Asylum Act, which has led to a sharp rise in the number of asylum seekers held in detention, despite having committed no criminal offence.

Inevitably, mental health is the single most important health problem affecting refugees, and it is important that medical staff should be aware of the patient's refugee background before diagnosis and treatment. Likewise, it is important for staff to be trained in refugee health. Currently, most health professionals in this country receive no formal training in this subject. Because of the unplanned, forced nature of their arrival in Britain, refugees come less prepared than other immigrants, and thus experience more difficulty in adjusting to life in the host country. Access to the health and social security systems, in particular, can be problematic because of language problems and unfamiliarity with British procedures. Advice and interpreting facilities are therefore of the utmost importance to ensure that refugees receive equal access to services.

Prior to the 1993 Asylum Act, over 75 per cent of those requesting asylum in Britain were granted temporary or permanent refugee status by the Home Office. Since the passing of the Act, however, the number of requests rejected by the Home Office has risen sharply: during the 12-month period after the Act was passed (July 1993) 74 per cent of requests for asylum were refused. The total number of refugee applications during 1993 was 22 370, and the figure for 1994 was 32 830. The increasing number of conflicts and political crises around the world, and the hardship arising from these situations, is likely to result in an ever-increasing number of applicants.

Further reading

Joly, D. & Nettleton, C. (1990) *Refugees in Europe.* Minority Rights Group, London.
Karmi, G. (1992) *Refugees and the National Health Service.* NE and NW Thames Regional Health Authorities, London.
Karmi, G. (1992) Refugee health. *British Medical Journal,* **305**, 205–6.
Migration and health in the 1990s. *International Migration Quarterly,* **30**, 1992.
Turner, S. (1989) Working with survivors. *Psychological Bulletin,* **13**, 173–6.

☎   National contacts

Jessica Judilovich, Kate Allen or
Julia Purcell
The Refugee Council
3 Bondway
London SW8 1SJ
Tel: 0171 582 6922

*The Medical Foundation for Care
of Victims of Torture*
96 Grafton Road
London NW5 3EJ
Tel: 0171 284 4321

Migrants Resource Centre
24 Churton Street
London SW1V 2LP
Tel: 0171 834 2505

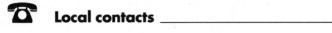 **Local contacts** _____

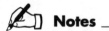 **Notes** _____

Part 2
Religions

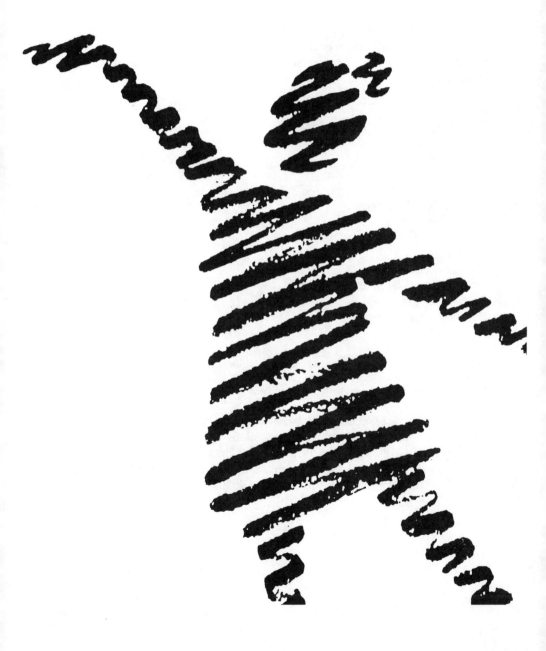

How to Use Part 2

The order of headings under each religion is as follows. The headings are only included if they are an issue for the ethnic group or particularly relevant to health care.

Languages[1]
Naming systems and titles[1]
Religious occasions and festivals
Religious obligations
Religious practices
Diet
Relevant social customs
Family planning
Birth
Death rites
Medical restrictions
Issues of particular interest
Further reading
National contacts and local contacts[2]
Notes[2]

[1] Only relevant in certain religions, where ethno-linguistic and religious identity are inter-changeable (in this case, Jews and Sikhs).
[2] Space has been left for the reader to add information.

Note: No separate section has been included for Christianity, although reference to different Christian denominations has been made in the text where relevant. This is because the majority of British doctors are assumed to be familiar with the basic beliefs of Christianity and also because there are, in general, no health implications to Christian rituals.

Buddhism

Buddhism is a way of life, incorporating a philosophy and a system of ethics, rather than a set of social rules. It revolves around a central tenet, that suffering can be stopped by eliminating selfish desires. Belief in rebirth encourages virtuous behaviour in this life, so that one may make spiritual progress in the next. The ultimate Buddhist goal is to escape the eternal cycle of life and death and reach a higher state of understanding and *Nirvana*. Buddhists are expected to observe five precepts (*silas*): do not kill; do not steal; maintain correct sexual contact; be truthful; and do not use intoxicating substances. Buddhism emphasises the importance of love for all living beings and respect for all forms of life, as well as charity, hospitality and self-discipline. There are many Buddhist sects, but the two main schools are *Mahayana*, prevalent in China and Japan, and *Therevada*, or 'Southern' Buddhism, prevalent in South East Asia. The latter school tends to be stricter in the interpretation of the original teachings of the Buddha, while *Mahayana* Buddhism has a more universal, popular approach.

Religious occasions and festivals

Sometime between April and May, at full moon, Buddhists throughout the world celebrate *Wesak*, which simultaneously marks the birth, enlightenment, and entry into *Parinirvana* (complete passing away) of the Buddha. *Wesak* also marks the Buddhist new year. Dates are based on a lunar calendar, and are therefore liable to vary. *Mahayana* Buddhists commemorate the same above events, but on three separate days, on 8 April, 8 December and 15 February respectively. They also celebrate *Ullumbana* (all souls) and new year.

Religious practices

Specific religious practices include observance of the five precepts (see above), *dana* (generosity, offering food to monks), meditation and chanting. Incense is often burned during meditation. Some Buddhists fast or abstain from eating meat on the first and fifteenth day of each lunar month, i.e. when the moon is either full or new. Pilgrimages to the four main sites relating to the life of Buddha are considered of great value. These are all located in India.

Diet

There are no specific dietary regulations, but most Buddhists are vegetarian.

Family planning

No specific regulations.

Death rites

Cremation is preferred. A monk or priest will normally officiate.

Medical restrictions

None.

Further reading

Cheetham, E. *Fundamentals of Mainstream Buddhism.* Available with other pamphlets from The Buddhist Society, London.
Shelling, J. (1987) *The Buddhist Handbook*. Rider, London.

☎ National contacts

Ron Maddox (General Secretary)
The Buddhist Society
58 Eccleston Square
London SW1 1PH
Tel: 0171 834 5858

London Buddhist Centre
51 Roman Road
London E2 0HU
Tel: 0181 981 1225

*Throssel Hole Priory (Mahayana/
Soto Zen)*
Carrshield
Hexham
Northumberland NE47 8AL
Tel: 01434 345204

*Amaravati Buddhist Monastery
(Therevada)*
Great Gaddesden
Hemel Hempstead
Hertfordshire HP1 3BZ
Tel: 01442 842455

☎ **Local contacts** _____

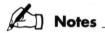 **Notes** _____

Hinduism

Hinduism is a social system as well as a set of religious beliefs; customs and religious practices are therefore closely interwoven. Religious practices vary a great deal, depending on caste and areas of origin. There is no single holy book equivalent to the Bible or Koran, although all true Hindus accept the *Bhagavaid Gita* as the most important script. Hindus worship many different gods, who are viewed as incarnations of a single superior being or Absolute Truth. Every Hindu is born into a caste which is determined by individual *karma* in a previous life. This reflects the central Hindu tenet of reward for good deeds and punishment for wickedness. Orthodox Hindus believe that a person's *karma* is permanent and cannot be altered, and disapprove of the mixing of castes through contact in any form. The caste system continues to exert a strong influence in Indian society, as well as among Indians in Britain, particularly when marriage partners are chosen.

Religious occasions and festivals

Major Hindu festivals are: *Mahashivaratri* (the birth of Shiva) in February or March, *Ram Navami* (birth of *Ram* and the incarnation of *Vishnu*) in March or April, *Janmastami* (the birth of *Krishna*) in August or September, and *Diwali*, the festival of light, in October. Dates vary slightly according to the cycle of the moon.

Religious obligations

Hindu rules vary according to caste. The higher the caste, the more religious observance is expected. The highest caste, *Brahmins*, have ultimate responsibility in religious matters. Fasting is usually done by devout Hindus, mainly by women. Some practising Hindus may fast regularly each week, depending on their loyalty to a particular deity or the astrological significance of certain days. Fasting in this sense implies eating only 'pure' foods such as fruits or yoghurt, rather than complete abstinence.

Religious practices

Every Hindu has a chosen god or *ishta devata*, and every home will have a prayer room (*puja*). Worship may take place anywhere, as God is considered omnipresent, however temple worship is customary, and a priest (*pujani*) may be in attendance to assist in rituals. Pictures and silver or gold idols of gods normally adorn the place of worship, and offerings (*arti*) are often made in the form of food or money.

Diet

The majority of Hindus do not eat meat, meat products (e.g. lard, gravy, etc.) or fish, and many abstain from eating eggs, as these are considered a potential source of life. Milk is always acceptable (although many South Asians are lactose-intolerant). Some lower caste Hindus eat meat but not beef, as cows are considered sacred. Pork is not usually eaten as pigs are regarded as unclean. Tea, coffee, garlic and onions are avoided by some Hindus because they are considered excessively stimulating. Alcohol is officially disapproved of, but not forbidden.

Relevant social customs

Spiritual purity and physical cleanliness are extremely important. Many Hindus prefer showers to baths. Modest dress is prescribed for men and women: men must be covered from waist to knees. Hindu women do not like to undress fully for medical examinations, and they also prefer to be examined by female medical staff.

Gold jewellery worn next to the skin is believed by many Hindus to ward off diseases. Thus, all items of jewellery may have personal, religious or cultural significance and are removed only reluctantly. Married women, for example, traditionally wear a *mangal sutra* or gold brooch given to them by their husbands or in-laws, as well as gold bangles. Men of the highest caste (*Brahmins*) may wear a sacred thread (*janeu*) over the right shoulder and around the body; its religious and cultural significance must be respected and it is removed with great reluctance. Men may wear other types of jewellery which have personal or religious significance and which they would be unwilling to remove. Married women traditionally wear small red spots or *bindi* on their foreheads, and some apply a stream of vermillion or *sindur* on the parting of their hair in the early years of marriage. Hindus prefer to wash themselves in running water, so showers are preferable to baths. As in other eastern religions, it is customary for people to remove footware on entering the home. Smoking is frowned upon but is not forbidden.

Family planning

There is no specific ruling about contraception. East African Hindus tend to be more willing to limit family size. Abortion is discouraged, but individual attitudes vary.

Birth

After birth, the mystical symbol *Om* (Supreme Spirit) is traditionally written in honey on the baby's tongue by a close relative. The baby's horoscope is also read and the birth is usually celebrated six or eleven days later. Traditional Hindu women do not leave the home for forty days after giving birth, and generally refrain from work during this period.

Death rites

Hindus are normally cremated. Post mortems are not prohibited, but some families consider them disrespectful.

Medical restrictions

Beef-derived insulin may be unacceptable.
Blood transfusions and organ transplants are permitted.

Issues of particular interest

Traditional medicine, such as *Ayurvedic* practice, usually operates alongside conventional health services. *Ayurvedic* practitioners are known as *vaidyas*. Diabetes and coronary heart disease have increased prevalence in all South Asian groups and more attention is being focused on the causes of this increased prevalence (see relevant ethnic groups).

Further reading

Henley, A. (1983) *Caring for Hindus and their families: religious aspects of care*. Asians in Britain Series. National Extension College/DHSS/ King's Fund Centre. National Extension College, Cambridge.
Karmi, G. (1995) *Traditional Asian Medicine in Britain*. MENAS Press, London.

McAvoy, B.R. & Donaldson, L.J. (1990) *Health Care for Asians.* Oxford
University Press, Oxford.

 National contacts _____

Mr Krishnamurthi or
Dr Nanda Kumar
*Bharatiya Vidya Bhavan (Institute
of Indian Arts and Culture)*
4a Castletown Road
London W14 9HQ
Tel: 0171 381 3086/381 4608

*Confederation of Indian
Organisations (UK)*
5 Westminster Bridge Road
London SE1 7XW
Tel: 0171 928 9889

India Welfare Society
11 Middle Row
London W10 5AT
Tel: 0181 969 9493

Mr Gopal Ghandi
*Cultural Section, Indian High
Commission*
India House
Aldwych
London WC2B 4NA
Tel: 0171 491 3567

Local contacts _____

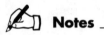 **Notes**

Islam

Followers of the Islamic faith are *Muslims*, meaning those who live their lives according to the will of *Allah* (God). Total submission to Allah is the central tenet of Islam, the rules of which are laid down in the Muslim holy book, the Koran. Islam is a practical religion, placing great emphasis on modesty, social responsibility, health, cleanliness, the importance of family ties and children. It recognises the importance of modern medicine, and there are few, if any, restrictions applied to medical procedures and practices. Even so, attitudes can vary according to the specific ethnic and socio-economic background of the patient. The two major sects of Islam are *Sunni* and *Shi'i*. There are some doctrinal differences between these two groups but their basic beliefs are predominantly the same. Most Muslims in the UK are from the Indian sub-continent, particularly Pakistan and Bangladesh.

Religious occasions and festivals

There are three main festivals: *Id al-Fitr* marks the end of the month of *Ramadan*, the fasting month. *Id al-Adha* (called *Bayram* by Turkish and Asian Muslims) marks the beginning of the *Hajj* or season of pilgrimage to Mecca. Muslims are obliged, circumstances and health permitting, to perform the pilgrimage once in their lifetime; *Mawlid al-Nabi* marks the birth of the Prophet Mohammad. Dates of festivals vary, as they are based on a lunar calendar. Friday is the Muslim holy day of rest.

Religious obligations

Adult Muslims are required to pray five times a day after ritual ablutions. The prayer sessions usually last for 10–15 minutes. Muslims are obliged to fast during the holy month of Ramadan, the ninth in the lunar calendar. In 1995 it ran from the 1–29 February. With each year, it comes forward by ten days on the Christian calendar, i.e. in 1996 Ramadan will be from 22 January to 19 February, and so on.

During Ramadan, the faithful must abstain from all food, drink, smoking and sexual activity between sunrise and sunset. Menstruating and pregnant women, pre-pubertal children, the sick and people on journeys are exempt from this obligation. Elderly people in poor health are partially or totally exempt. Many people choose to fast, even though they qualify for exemption. This can cause problems for diabetics and those suffering from gastric ulcers. Some pious Muslims will refuse injections or even eye-drops during Ramadan, although there are no religious rulings against this.

Diet

Eating pork in any form is forbidden in Islam. In this connection, it is important for medical staff to consult the patient before prescribing pork-derived insulin. Other meat may be eaten, provided it is *halal*, that is killed in the manner prescribed by Islamic law, i.e. by severing the animal's jugular vein to allow the blood to drain out of the body. Fish is acceptable providing it has scales (i.e. no swordfish, eel, shark, etc.). The consumption of alcohol in any form is prohibited.

Muslims are required to fast from dawn to dusk during the holy month of Ramadan (see 'Religious obligations').

Relevant social customs

Except for close family members, men and women are normally segregated to varying degrees, depending on the strength of adherence to tradition. Pre- and extra-marital relations are prohibited. Great importance is attached to bridal virginity. Both men and women are required to dress modestly. Nakedness is considered shameful. Patients almost invariably prefer to be examined by a doctor of their own sex.

All Muslim boys are circumcised before puberty. Muslims from India and Pakistan prefer circumcision to take place a few days after birth, whereas Bangladeshi families may postpone the event for up to eight years. Circumcision is considered a major life-event, and is often celebrated with enthusiasm. In rural areas the operation is traditionally performed by a local barber if no doctor is available. Hospitals in Britain do not always carry out free circumcisions on the grounds that they are medically unnecessary. The decision whether to charge patients for the operation currently rests with individual hospitals.

Some jewellery may hold cultural or economic significance. The bride is traditionally given gold jewellery as part of her dowry, and it is removed reluctantly.

It is customary for Muslims to remove shoes at the entrance to the home, and use separate footwear in the toilet. There is also a preference for showers instead of baths, as running water is considered essential for cleanliness. It is customary for Muslims to wash with running water the private parts of their bodies after toilet use.

Some observant Muslims tend to avoid using the left hand, especially when handling food, or when passing something to someone.

Family planning

There is no specific Islamic ruling against contraception. Nevertheless it is disapproved of by custom. Similarly, abortion is frowned upon, but often tolerated for medical reasons.

Death rites

The body should be buried as soon as possible after death. It is washed, and wrapped in a white cotton or linen cloth. Following a religious ceremony, the body is buried directly in the earth, facing Mecca, without a coffin. Cremations are not permitted. Post mortems are forbidden unless absolutely necessary.

Medical restrictions

Medical needs are given priority; therefore restrictions are minimal. There are no specific rulings prohibiting blood transfusions or organ transplants.

Issues of particular interest

Some Muslim communities, particularly North Africans, may use traditional healers or *faqihs*, and traditional medicines alongside conventional treatment. It should be pointed out that there are many cultural differences between Muslims from different parts of the Islamic world. For example, the wearing of the veil (*hijab, chador*), is not practised by all Muslims to the same degree: some women cover the entire body, while others just wear a headscarf or none at all.

For details on female circumcision, which is often mistakenly associated with Islam, see under 'Somalis'.

Further reading

Chippendale, P. & Horrie, C. (1990) *What is Islam?* Virgin, London.

Guillaume, A. (1990) *Islam.* Penguin, London.

Henley, A. (1982) *Caring for Muslims and their families: religious aspects of care.* Asians in Britain Series. National Extension College/DHSS/King's Fund Centre. National Extension College, Cambridge.

Lewis, P. (1994) *Islamic Britain.* I.B. Tauris, London.

National contacts _____

Dr Zaki Badawi
Moulana Shahid Raza
The Muslim College
20–22 Creffield Road
Ealing
London W5 3RP
Tel: 0181 992 6636

Mr Bashir
Islamic Cultural Centre
London Central Mosque (Regent's Park)
146 Park Road
London NW8 7RG
Tel: 0171 724 3363

*Islamic Universal Foundation
(Shi'ia Mosque)*
20 Penzance Place
Holland Park
London W11 4PG
Tel: 0171 602 5273

 Local contacts _____

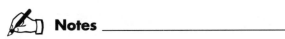

Notes

Judaism

The Jewish community considers itself both a religious and an ethnic group. Although there has been an indigenous Jewish population in Britain from the Middle Ages onwards, most British Jews are descended from migrants who came to Britain from Eastern and Central Europe during the 19th and early 20th centuries. Others came as refugees from Nazi persecution during and after the Second World War. Broadly, Jews can be divided into two ethnic sub-groups: *Ashkenazi* Jews, who originate from Eastern and Central Europe, and *Sephardi* Jews, who came from Spain, North Africa and the Middle East. The Jewish community in Britain is very diverse, reflecting differing degrees of assimilation, religious observance, and geographical origin. There is a strong emphasis on family ties throughout the Jewish community, especially among the observant. Many Jews in Britain have a high standard of education, and hold professional occupations. The community is generally well provided with organisations that care for elderly and disadvantaged groups.

There are Jewish communities all over Britain, mainly in large towns. Orthodox Jews are concentrated in the districts of Golders Green, Finchley and Stamford Hill in North London. There is also a sizeable Jewish community in Lancashire, notably in Manchester.

Languages

English is almost universally spoken. Yiddish is spoken by some of the elderly and by members of the Orthodox religious community, the *Haredim* (*Hassidim*, *Sephardim* and *Misnagdim*) and the *Lubavitch* sect. Hebrew is the language of prayer (and of Israelis). Other languages such as Polish or German are also spoken, depending on the area of origin. Jews from North Africa and parts of the Middle East use Arabic.

Religious occasions and festivals

Among the most important annual events are *Rosh Hashanah* (New Year), also known as *Yom ha-Din* (Judgement Day), in September/October and *Yom Kippur* (the Day of Atonement), which takes place ten days later. In early spring there is *Pesach* (Passover) which celebrates the exodus from Egypt, followed by the harvest festival *Shavuot* (Pentecost) fifty days later. *Sukkot* (Tabernacles) is the autumn harvest festival. There are several other minor feast days and fasts throughout the year, among them *Chanukah* or *Hannukah*, an eight-day event in mid-December marked by lighting candles, and *Purim* (the story of Esther). Saturday is the weekly day of rest (see 'Religious obligations').

These events are based on the lunar calendar, so dates vary from year to year.

Religious obligations

Jewish religious practices are laid down in the *Torah* (the first five books of the Bible), and interpreted by the rabbis or religious teachers in the *Talmud* and other religious texts. Orthodox Jews observe these teachings strictly, while others, such as the Progressive, Reform and Liberal groups, make more concessions to modern lifestyles. Many Jews have abandoned ritual practice altogether. Virtually all ritual laws are waived if life is considered to be in danger.

The Sabbath (*Shabbat*), the Day of Rest, begins at sunset on Friday and ends on Saturday evening. On the Sabbath, Orthodox Jews will not do any type of work, or physical activities, including relatively small tasks, such as carrying a bag, driving, switching a light on or pushing a pram.

Fasting occurs for 25 hours, beginning at sunset on the eve of *Yom Kippur*. Orthodox patients must be offered alternatives to oral medication, such as injections or suppositories. For them this day is emotional and highly significant. Some patients also observe the fast of *Tisha B'av* with equal strictness.

Nearly all Jewish boys are circumcised, usually eight days after birth; only a qualified *mohel* is accepted by the Orthodox to carry out this operation. A clotting disorder of the blood, e.g. haemophilia, usually disqualifies a man for circumcision, as mentioned in the *Talmud* in c. AD 500 (the first known reference to this condition). A *mohel* should be consulted on all religious matters. Infant jaundice will also delay circumcision until the child has recovered. At the age of 13, boys are accepted as full members of the community in a ceremony known as *Bar Mitzvah*. There is a corresponding ceremony, known as *Bat Mitzvah*, for Orthodox girls held at the age of 12.

Modesty in dress is an important religious issue for practising Jews. Orthodox men keep their heads covered with a hat or skull cap (*kappel*), and the strictly religious wear a four-fringed undergarment (*tallit katan*) during the day. Many women cover their hair in public with a scarf or a wig (*scheitel*), while some *Haredim* men will not shake hands with women, even preferring not to look at them or speak to them.

Diet

Dietary regulations are observed to varying degrees by all practising Jews. Pork and its derivatives and shellfish are *treifa*, i.e. strictly prohibited. Other meat is *kosher* (permitted) provided it has been slaughtered according to Jewish law. Orthodox Jews are not permitted to eat meat and dairy products together or within several hours of each other, and must use separate plates and utensils for them; but practice varies. Separate kitchens may be maintained by wealthier families. Practising Jews are not supposed to take non-*kosher* medication unless there are no alternatives; in this case they must be instructed to do so specifically by the doctor and by a rabbi. All food has to be specially inspected by a rabbi (except fruit and vegetables), and bears a special label to show that it has been passed.

For the eight days of *Pesach* no leavened bread or cakes or biscuits are eaten. Some medicines may also be forbidden, and special advice from the rabbi will be required by health professionals. During Passover Orthodox Jews will not eat *any* food unless specifically supervised.

Family planning

Some Orthodox Jews forbid contraception and abortion unless the mother's health is at risk. There are no specific guidelines relating to infertility/fertility treatment. However, rabbinic consultation is advisable.

Death rites

Funeral services are relatively simple. Preferably the body must be interred within 24 hours of death. Progressive Jews allow cremation, although it is forbidden by Jewish law. Post mortems are not permitted unless legally required. Following the funeral, close relatives remain at home and refrain from daily activities. During this period of mourning (*shivah*) services take place in the home and relatives and friends will bring in food.

Medical restrictions

Blood transfusions are permitted. Organ transplants are usually forbidden by Orthodox Jews. However, opinions vary, and decisions may rest with the rabbinic authority.

Issues of particular interest

A small number of Jews are Hassidic, belonging to an ultra-Orthodox movement which originated in 18th-century Poland. Men and boys traditionally dress in black and grow distinctive locks (*payot*) on the sides of their heads. As this group is characterised by strict religious observance and restrictions on outside contacts, the Hassidic rabbi may need to be consulted before any medical intervention. The Hassidic community maintains its own Hebrew schools and literacy or fluency in English among pupils attending these schools may be reduced. Making contact with this group can be difficult because of their reluctance to interact socially with outsiders.

The diet of many Orthodox Jews is high in carbohydrates and contains little fresh fruit and vegetables. As a result, general nutrition is often poor.

Tay-Sachs disease, a severe genetic disorder of early childhood which is invariably fatal, is a characteristic of *Ashkenazi* Jews.

Further reading

Close, B.E. (1993) *Judaism*. Hodder and Stoughton, London.
Cross, C. (1974) *What is Judaism?* Board of Deputies of British Jews, London.
Lancaster, B. (1993) *The Elements of Judaism*. Element, London.

☎ National contacts

Esme Daniels, Educational Consultant
Board of Deputies of British Jews
Woburn House
Upper Woburn Place
London WC1H 0EP
Tel: 0171 387 3952

Evan Millner, Jewish Programmes Director
Jewish Care
221 Golders Green Road
London NW11 9DW
Tel: 0181 458 3282 ext. 226

For information on burials and circumcisions:
Beth Din (Office of the Chief Rabbi)
Alder House
Tavistock Square
London WC1H 9HN
Tel: 0171 387 1066

The Hillel Foundation
25 Louisa Street
London E1 1BA
Tel: 0171 790 5426

**For further information on the
Hassidic community:**
Union of Hebrew Congregations
40 Queen Elizabeth's Walk
London N16 0HH
Tel: 0181 802 6226

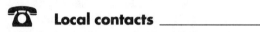 **Local contacts**

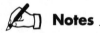 **Notes**

Sikhism

The Sikh community is both an ethnic and a religious group. Founded by Guru Nanak in the 16th century, the Sikh faith has its roots in Hinduism, but developed into a separate religion over the course of the following 200 years. Unlike Hindus, Sikhs are monotheistic, worshipping one supreme God, and believe in the equality of all before the creator. However, certain beliefs are shared with Hinduism, notably belief in reincarnation and *karma*. Religious life revolves around the *gurdwara*, or Sikh temple. The Sikh community is divided into two categories of believers: the *Saihajdharis*, who are apprentices and the *Amridharis* who have been formally baptised. The latter have to abide by a strict code of dress and the wearing of signs of Sikh identity.

Sikhism has always been inextricably bound up with the language, culture and history of the Punjab, in North West India, where 90 per cent of India's Sikhs live and where most Sikhs in Britain originate from (see also 'Punjabis – Pakistanis').

Languages

The mother tongue of the Sikh community is Punjabi, which is written in the *gurmukhi* script.

Naming systems and titles

Most Sikhs have three names: a first name, a religious title (*Singh*, meaning lion, for all men and *Kaur*, meaning 'prince' for all women), and a family name. (The title 'prince' was originally bestowed on women in an attempt to bring their status closer to that of men. However, the word is generally translated as 'princess' to avoid confusion.) The family name is not used by devout Sikhs, since family names can often imply caste or sub-caste, which Sikhism does not accept. In Britain family names are sometimes used to ease administrative procedures. The accepted form of address is to use the first name followed by *Singh* for a man, e.g. Mr Amarjit Singh. Similarly, a woman's first name should always be followed by *Kaur*, omitting the family surname.

It should be noted that some Hindus born in Rajastan also use the name *Singh*, without any Sikh religious connotations, as a family surname.

Religious occasions and festivals

The main Sikh festivals are *Vaisakhi* (New Year) on 13 April; *Diwali*, held in October/November; and *Hola*, a three-day pageant in February or March. The most important commemorative occasions (*gurpurbs*) are the birthday of the founder of Sikhism, Guru Nanak, and the birthday of Guru Gobind Singh, the most revered Sikh warrior and hero. Other important anniversaries include the martyrdom of Guru Arjan and Guru Tegh Bahadur. All these days vary according to the phases of the moon.

For practical reasons, Sunday is the day of collective worship among Sikhs in Britain.

Religious obligations

Formally baptised Sikh men (*Amridharis*) wear the five signs of Sikhism, known as the five Ks: *kesh* (uncut hair), *kangha* (comb), *kara* (steel bangle), *kirpan* (symbolic dagger) and *kaccha* (symbolic undershorts). A turban (*pagri*), the most visible badge of Sikh identity, must be worn by all Sikh men, and only a small minority of Sikhs in Britain do not wear one. Long hair is worn in a bun and covered by a *rumal* or *patka* (inner turban) in some cases. The *kara* is an important talisman and is removed with the greatest reluctance. Many devout Sikhs always wear a *kaccha*, even if only round one leg, and some may refuse to undress completely for medical examination. Many Sikhs in Britain have chosen to give up some of the five Ks, but the devout are reluctant to remove any of them at any time. Sikh women usually cover their hair with a scarf (*dupatta*) or, in a few cases, with a tight black or white turban.

Smoking is strictly forbidden.

Diet

Although meat is not specifically prohibited, many observant Sikhs are vegetarian and do not eat fish or eggs (more women than men are vegetarian within the Sikh community in Britain). Meat has to be *jhatka* or *chakar*, i.e. slaughtered with one stroke. Eating meat according to the *halal* or *kosher* method of draining all blood from the animal (see 'Islam' and 'Judaism') is strictly prohibited. Some Sikhs, particularly those who have lived with Hindu populations, may avoid eating beef, as cows are respected animals in India. Pork is generally avoided, as it is considered unclean.

Some devout Sikhs eat only certain foods, such as fruits, on a given day; this is a matter of personal choice.

Intoxicants are officially discouraged, although many Sikh men drink alcohol (see 'Issues of particular interest').

Relevant social customs

Traditional dress for men is the pajama and *kameez* or *kurta* (long buttoned shirt with a high collar), and the *shalwar kameez* for women. Married women dislike removing their wedding bangles or wedding rings, unless their husbands have died. Female patients prefer to consult a female doctor, as modesty is important.

Generally speaking, Sikhs prefer to wash in running water, in the shower rather than in the bath.

(See also 'Religious obligations'.)

Family planning

There are no specific religious prohibitions against contraception, but large families are traditionally regarded as desirable. Abortion is frowned on and only permitted in extreme cases.

Birth

It is customary for mothers to be given rich foods following childbirth. The event is celebrated by thanksgiving at the *gurdwara* (temple). Among traditional Sikhs, mothers are not allowed to cook for forty days after childbirth.

Death rites

The family is responsible for all ceremonies and rites at death. There are usually no objections to the body being tended by non-Sikhs, but close consultation with the family is essential on all matters of procedure. Sikhs are cremated, if possible within 24 hours of death, and the ashes are scattered in running water.

Medical restrictions

Post mortems, blood transfusions and organ transplants are permitted.

Issues of particular interest

As in all South Asian groups, the incidence of diabetes and coronary heart disease in the group is high. There are also indications that alcoholism among Sikh men is more common than among other South Asian groups, although it is still less common than among white British males. Members of this community use traditional *Ayurvedic* medicine, and consult traditional healers (*Vaids*). Health professionals need to be aware of this, in order to guard against dual therapy and drug interaction.

Further reading

Bhachu, P. (1985) *Twice Migrants. East African Sikh Settlers in Britain*. Tavistock, London.
Henley, A. (1983) *Caring for Sikhs and their families: religious aspects of care*. Asians in Britain Series. National Extension College/DHSS/King's Fund Centre. National Extension College, Cambridge.
McAvoy, B.R. & Donaldson, L.J. (1990) *Health Care for Asians*. Oxford University Press, Oxford.

 National contacts

Professor Harminder Singh
Sikh Divine Fellowship
46 Sudbury Court Drive
Harrow
Middlesex UB6 0NR
Tel: 0181 904 9244

Sikh Missionary Resource Centre
346 Green Lane
Small Heath
Birmingham B9 5DR
Tel: 0121 7725365

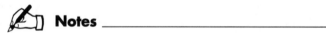 **Local contacts** _____

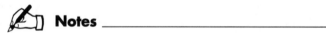 **Notes** _____

Part 3
Ethnic Groups

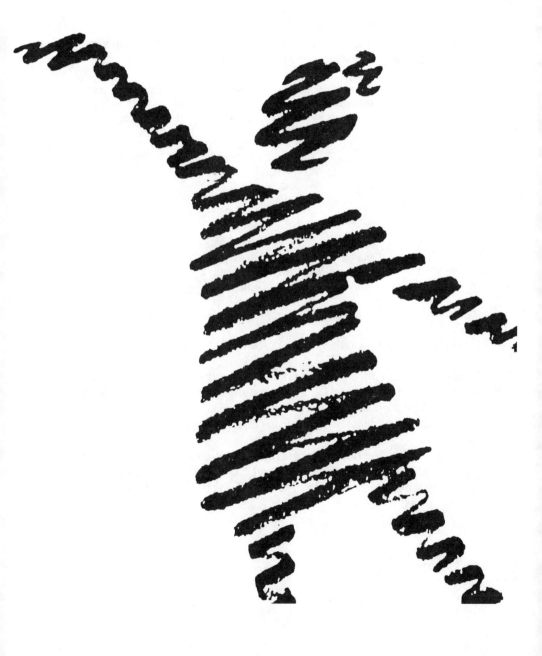

How to Use Part 3

The reader will not find the following ethnic groups under their own separate headings. Instead, please refer to the sections indicated.

Africans*	see Eritreans Ethiopians Ghanaians Nigerians Somalis Sudanese	Gypsies	see Traveller-Gypsies
		Indians	see Hinduism Sikhism Gujaratis Punjabis – Pakistanis Tamils
Asians	see Hinduism Islam Sikhism Bangladeshis Gujaratis Punjabis – Pakistanis Tamils	North Africans (Algerians, Egyptians, Libyans, Moroccans and Tunisians)	see Arabs
Bengalis	see Bangladeshis	Rastafarians	see African-Caribbeans
Greeks	see Cypriots – Greek	Turkish	see Cypriots – Turkish

*The majority of Africans in Britain come from the West African Commonwealth states of Nigeria and Ghana. Other important groups include Somalis, Eritreans, Sudanese and Kenyans, but the list also includes small numbers of Botswanans, Ugandans, South Africans and Ethiopians, and is by no means exhaustive.

It is important for health professionals to be aware that there is a high prevalence of AIDS in certain East and Central African countries. These groups have not been included in *The Handbook* because numbers in Britain are very small.

The order of headings under each ethnic group is as follows. The headings are only included if they are an issue for the ethnic group, or particularly relevant to health care.

Languages
Naming systems and titles
Religion
Customs and relevant religious practices
Festivals and holy days
Dress
Diet
Birth
Death rites
Social customs
Family planning
Medical restrictions
Specific health issues
Further reading
National contacts and local contacts*
Notes*

* Space has been left for the reader to add information.

African-Caribbeans

The term African-Caribbean (or Afro-Caribbean) describes people of African origin who came to Britain from the Caribbean islands, notably Jamaica, Trinidad and Tobago, Grenada, Dominica, Barbados, St Lucia and the British Virgin Islands. There have been people from the Caribbean in Britain since the 17th century, but the majority of migrants were invited to Britain during the 1950s and early 1960s in response to a shortage of manual labour. The majority of African-Caribbeans live in urban areas, mainly in London, the West Midlands, Bristol, and in Lancashire.

People of Caribbean origin in Britain face economic hardship and social deprivation, in which racism often plays a part.

Languages

English is universally spoken and written, but many people speak a dialect or *patois*, which combines elements of English, Western European and African languages.

Religion

Most African-Caribbeans are mainstream Christians. Within this group there are well-defined groups of Pentacostalists, Seventh Day Adventists, and Jehovah's Witnesses. A smaller number are Baptists, Anglicans, Methodists or Roman Catholics. An increasing proportion, particularly among the young, are Rastafarians, or are influenced by them.

The Rastafarian movement, which gained prominence in the 1920s and 1930s as an extension of the Marcus Garvey movement, is millenarian in outlook, i.e. its followers await a messiah. They feel that they are being held captive in the Western World, which they call Babylon, and look to Africa for redemption. There is no clearly defined Rastafarian ideology, but central to the movement is the veneration of the late Emperor of Ethiopia, Haile Salassie I, the 'Lion of Judah', and the Messiah of the Black race, who was known as Ras Tafari before his coronation in 1930. Rastafarians in the Caribbean rejected the European orientation of Caribbean culture, and also the various Christian revivalist movements. The movement expanded in the

1960s, in parallel with the upsurge of Black consciousness and the US civil rights movements in general.

Diet

Most Seventh Day Adventists avoid pork and pork products. Some do not drink tea or coffee, because they are regarded as excessively stimulating. Many Rastafarians also avoid pork; others are vegetarians and refuse to eat grape products; some refuse to use salt. Some Rastafarians are vegans and many avoid foods containing additives and preservatives.

Social customs

Rastafarians wear their hair long, in so-called 'dread-locks', which are never combed or cut, but instead tidied with olive oil or coconut oil. *Ganja* (marijuana) is commonly smoked for religious purposes and on social occasions, especially among the young.

Family planning

Many Rastafarians oppose contraception because past family planning programmes in the Caribbean were viewed as racist. Abortion is considered repugnant by many African-Caribbean women.

Medical restrictions

Jehovah's Witnesses are opposed to blood transfusions.

Specific health issues

Sickle cell disease is a cardinal feature in this community.

The incidence of hypertension and stroke is raised among African-Caribbeans in Britain, as is also that of diabetes.

G6PD deficiency is present (see page 63). Certain drugs can cause haemolysis, e.g. anti-malarials and sulphonamides. For further details please refer to the British National Formulary (BNF).

A strikingly elevated rate of psychiatric hospital admission of African-Caribbeans for schizophrenia has been noted, especially among the second generation British-born African-Caribbeans. The reasons for this high admission rate are still unclear, though the lower prevalence of schizophrenia in the Caribbean and among first generation migrants points towards factors related to migration and life in Britain as a possible explanation.

Further reading

Balarajan, R. (1991) Ethnic differences in mortality from ischaemic heart disease and cerebrovascular disease in England and Wales. *British Medical Journal*, **302**, 560–64.
Cruickshank, J.K. & Beevers, D.G. (1989) *Ethnic Factors in Health and Disease*. Chapters 12–15; 22; 33–5. Butterworth-Heinemann, Guildford.
Kaplan, N.M. (1994) Ethnic aspects of hypertension. *Lancet*, **344**, 450–52.
Littlewood, R. & Lipsedge, M. (1988) Psychiatric illness among British Afro-Caribbeans. *British Medical Journal*, **296**, 950–51.

☎ National contacts

African-Caribbean Community Development Unit (ACCDU)
London Voluntary Sector Resource Centre
356 Holloway Road
London N7 6PN
Tel: 0171 700 8148

Afro-Caribbean Mental Health Association (ACMHA)
35–37 Electric Avenue
Brixton
London SW9 8JP
Tel: 0171 737 3603

Ian Mello
Afro-Caribbean Mental Health Project
Zion Community Health and Resource Centre
Zion Crescent
Hulme
Manchester M15 5BY
Tel: 0161 226 9562

Karl Smith
Health Care Advisor
(Health and Race)
Liverpool Health Authority
Hamilton House
24 Pall Mall
Liverpool L3 6AL
Tel: 0151 709 3181

Sickle Cell Society
54 Station Road
Harlesden
London NW10 4UX
Tel: 0181 961 7795

Thalassaemia and Sickle Cell Clinic
Ladywood Health Centre
395 Ladywood Middleway
Birmingham B16 2TP
Tel: 0121 454 4262

Veronica Campbell
*Bradford West Indian Community
Association*
Check Point Centre
45 Westgate
Bradford BD1 2RO
Tel: 01274 722996

*West Indian Family Counselling
Service*
Roscoe Methodist Church
Francis Street
Leeds LS7 4BY
Tel: 0113 262 5131

 Local contacts _____

 Notes _____

Arabs

'Arab' is the generic term applied to inhabitants of the Middle East and North Africa whose mother tongue is Arabic and who are, for the most part, either Muslims or identify with Islamic culture (see 'Islam'). Arabs in Britain come mainly from Egypt, the Gulf States, Iraq, Lebanon, Libya, Morocco, Palestine, Sudan, Somalia and Yemen. There are also smaller communities of Algerians, Omanis, Jordanians and Syrians. The overwhelming majority of these are concentrated in London, but there are other areas where Arab communities live, notably in Birmingham, Cardiff, Tyneside (Yemenis) and Manchester (Syrians). Generally speaking, the Arabs are less permanently settled in Britain than most other groups, and do not view themselves as an immigrant group. The one notable exception is the Yemenis, who originally settled in Britain as shipworkers in the 1870s, and are well-integrated.

Contrary to the popular notion of 'the wealthy Arab', which applies mainly to a small number of people – mainly visitors from Saudi Arabia and the Gulf States – a large proportion of Arabs are here as political exiles and refugees (most Sudanese, Lebanese, Somalis and Iraqis), or as migrant labourers. The Moroccan community, for example, consists almost entirely of migrant workers in the hotel and catering industry, many of whom support extended families in their home country.

Languages

Arabic is spoken in a range of dialects and accents, depending on country of origin, but all literate Arabs understand, read and write Modern Standard Arabic based on Classical Arabic, the language of the *Qur'an* (Koran). North Africans (Moroccans and Algerians) may also speak French, Berber and Spanish. Many Arabs resident in Britain speak English as a second language. However, because they are relative newcomers, and do not intend to stay in Britain long-term, Arabs often face difficulties in understanding everday English, and have little incentive to learn the language thoroughly.

Naming systems and titles

Arabic first names are often Islamic, and may be indistinguishable from the names of Pakistanis, Bangladeshis and other Muslim groups. Examples include Ali, Muhammad, Omar, Fatima, Ayesha. Other commonly-encountered male religious names are prefixed by Abdul, e.g. Abdul-Rahman, Abdul-Aziz. Also typical is the ending 'i', e.g. Hashemi, Husseini, Tabari. Arabic first names may also be non-Islamic, for example: Amir, Nadia, Rana.

Religion

The vast majority of Arabs are Muslim (see 'Islam'). A minority of Lebanese, Palestinians and Iraqis and Syrians are Christians, as are the Copts in Egypt. The Coptic Church is an ancient branch of Orthodox Christianity that developed in the Nile Valley. Palestinian and Iraqi Christians are Protestant, Catholic or Greek Orthodox, while the majority of Lebanese Christians belong to the Maronite Church founded by St Maroun in the 5th century.

Customs and relevant religious practices

The extent of religious practice varies from one individual to another. Women from the Gulf States often wear a full *hijab* (veil), covering most of the face, whereas Moroccan women may only wear a scarf over their heads.

Social values such as generosity and hospitality are held in high esteem. Gender roles among Arabs tend to be very clearly defined, and family ties are considered of the utmost importance. Traditionally, Muslim Arabs marry very young, although this is changing. It is customary for people from the Gulf States to use kohl, a black cosmetic powder, on the eyes of very young children. This can be toxic, as some varieties of kohl contain lead or, rarely, antimony.

(See also 'Islam'.)

Specific health issues

Because of the higher rate of consanguineous marriage among Muslims, the risk of hereditary disorders tends to be greater in this group.

Diabetes is relatively common, especially among Gulf Arabs and Moroccans.

Thalassaemia is particularly prevalent among Arabs from the Mediterranean region (North Africans, Lebanese, Palestinians and Syrians).

There is also a raised incidence of haemophilia among Gulf Arabs. Some Arab groups, notably Moroccans and Sudanese, practise traditional herbal medicine for minor ailments.

Many Palestinians, Lebanese and Iraqis resident in Britain are refugees. Consequently, they often suffer from stress, trauma and anxiety as their future, and that of their families from whom many are separated, is uncertain.

Iraqis, Libyans and Syrians have at various times been under threat of persecution by their own security services.

Further reading

El Solh, F.C. (1992) Arab communities in Britain: cleavages and commonality. In: *Islam and Christian-Muslim Relations*, **3** (2), 237–57.
Halliday, F. (1992) *Arabs in Exile*. I.B. Tauris, London.

 National contacts _____

Moroccan Information and Advice Centre
61 Golborne Road
London W10 5NR
Tel: 0181 960 6672

The Arab Club of Great Britain
1 St Dunstan's Avenue
London W3 6QD
Tel: 0181 992 4916

(See also 'Islam'.)

Emad Salman
Iraqi Community Association
Palingswick House
241 King Street
London W6 9LP
Tel: 0181 741 5491

 Local contacts _____

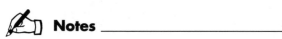 **Notes**

Armenians

Armenians first came to Britain as refugees after the First World War, following Turkish persecution between 1895 and 1920 under the Ottoman Empire. The second wave of refugees came to Britain from the Middle East, from countries such as Cyprus, Lebanon, Syria, Iraq, Iran and Turkey: political and social upheavals in these countries over the last 20 years have prompted large-scale movements of Armenians towards Western Europe and the United States. Many of these refugees and immigrants have experienced trauma before arriving in Britain, and may feel isolated because of the unfamiliarity of the language and culture in their new surroundings. The Armenian homeland remains divided today between Iran, Turkey and the former Soviet Republic of Armenia, now independent. Recent ethnic conflict and economic hardship has brought a further number of Armenians to seek safety and better opportunities in the West.

The British Armenian community is concentrated in West London, particularly in the borough of Ealing.

Languages

In addition to Armenian, these people often speak the language of the country they were born in, for example, Arabic, Persian, Turkish, Russian. Armenians from Iran and the former Soviet Union speak the Eastern Armenian dialect, while those from other parts of the Middle East and Europe speak the Western dialect. Armenian uses a unique alphabet, dating back to AD 406.

Naming systems and titles

All Armenian names (except when westernised) end in 'ian' meaning 'son of': hence, Manoukian, Kachatourian, Abrahamian.

Religion

Armenians are Christians, belonging to the Armenian Apostolic Church.

Festivals and holy days

Zadic or Easter Day on 15 April, and *Sourp Znnount*, the Epiphany, on 6 January, are the most important religious occasions. It is customary not to eat meat during the Easter period.

Social customs

Children must be baptised in order to be accepted as part of the community. Armenians have a strong sense of cultural identity and family ties.

Specific health issues

Thalassaemia is a feature in this group.

Many recently arrived refugees suffer from insecurity and culture-shock. However, as a result of previous experiences of persecution and mass-migration, the Armenians have a relatively well-organised network of groups offering care and assistance in host countries.

Further reading

No major references for this group are available.

☎ National contacts

Misak Ohanian, General Secretary
Centre for Armenian Information and Advice
105a Mill Hill Road
Acton
London W3 8JF
Tel: 0181 993 8953

Archbishop Yegishe Gizirian
Armenian Apostolic Oriental Orthodox Church
St Peter's Church
Cranley Gardens
London SW7 3BB
Tel: 0171 937 0152

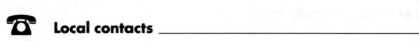

☎ **Local contacts** _____

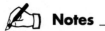 **Notes** _____

Bangladeshis

Like many other ethnic minorities, Bangladeshis mostly migrated to Britain for economic reasons. A large proportion of families come from the rural tea-growing region of Sylhet in North Eastern Bangladesh. Bengali men began to migrate to Britain in the 1940s, with arrivals reaching a peak in the 1960s and 1970s. Thereafter, most Bangladeshi migrants were women and children, as tighter immigration rules prevented men from travelling regularly to Bangladesh to visit their families. About half the Bangladeshi community in Britain is concentrated in the Borough of Tower Hamlets in the East End of London. The remainder are largely settled in the borough of Camden, and in the North of England.

One of the most important barriers to improving the health of the Bangladeshi community is language. Although members of the community have strong faith in modern medicine and consult doctors frequently, treatment is often followed incorrectly or left incomplete due to poor understanding of English, unfamiliarity with prescriptions, and the patient's own traditional health beliefs. Faith healing is commonly practised for both physical and mental illnesses alongside conventional medicine.

Languages

The three most commonly spoken languages are Sylheti, English and Bengali and some speak Urdu. Sylheti is a dialect of Bengali and is not written. Those who had access to education in Bangladesh read and write standard Bengali, which uses the Arabic script. Relatively few people in the community speak and write English fluently, and many do not speak English at all. Women seldom go out alone, and so have little opportunity to learn English. Many of the health problems of this community could be alleviated by effective communication between health providers and patients. This requires professional interpreting and regular follow-up to ensure that instructions are being followed.

Naming systems and titles

Men and women have different naming systems. Men traditionally have two or three names: a personal and a religious name, and a last name which may be a male title or an extended family (clan) name, such as Khan or Chowdhuri. The use of the surname is optional. In some cases a father's personal name may have been adopted as a British-style surname for administrative purposes in Britain, as individual family surnames are not used in Bangladesh. An example of a man's name is Muhammad (religious name), Yunus (personal name), Khan (clan name). The personal name comes either first or second.

Women usually have two names: a personal name such as Amina or Nadia followed by a female title such as Bibi, Begum, Khanum, Khatoon or Kausar. The title is meaningless on its own; Miss or Mrs Bibi is not acceptable, nor is Mrs Begum. A few women also use their husband's or father's name as a surname. Passports may be the only reliable documents showing correct name, spelling and date of birth. Even then, the last is often inaccurate.

Religion

The majority of Bangladeshis are *Sunni* Muslims (see 'Islam'). There are also significant Shia Muslim, Hindu, Christian and Buddhist minorities.

Customs and relevant religious practices

See 'Islam'.

Dress

The traditional dress of Bangladeshi women is the *sari* worn over a waist-length blouse and a long underskirt. The head is usually covered by the *sari* or a headscarf (*burka/hijab*). Young women wear *shalwar kameez* (long shirt over loose trousers) and/or baggy western dress. Older, devout men wear a skullcap sometimes together with a *kameez* (a long shirt) and *pajama* (baggy trousers).

Diet

The traditional Bengali diet is healthy, being rich in fish, vegetables, and pulses. Problems arise in Britain, when dietary customs change, notably to a higher sugar and lower fibre intake. This results in more dental decay, especially in children, and may well contribute to poorer general health.

For dietary restrictions see 'Islam'.

Social customs

Chewing *pan* is a very common custom in Bengali society and is practised by men and women. *Pan* is a mixture of lime betel leaves, betel nuts and other nuts and grains, and is usually eaten after meals. Adults often combine the above mixture with tobacco leaves. The ingredients are often grown at home, so *pan* is available easily and cheaply. When chewed, the mixture turns a brilliant red colour; this is considered attractive on the lips of young women. However, *pan* is associated with a number of health risks. The betel nut is the subject of ongoing research; it is addictive and can cause dizziness and per-spiration; it may also be linked to diabetes. Chewing tobacco has the added risk of cancer of the mouth, throat and stomach.

Heavy cigarette smoking, which is common among men, and is increasing among women, may be linked to a higher reported prevalence of duodenal ulcers in this group.

Specific health issues

The incidence of tuberculosis (TB), especially the extra-pulmonary type, is high in this group. This may be linked to infection and reinfection from travel to Bangladesh, where TB is endemic, and to low socio-economic status.

As is the case for other South Asian groups, there is an increased incidence of coronary heart disease and diabetes.

Peptic ulcer is particularly common in Bangladeshi men and current research is directed at investigating the cause, which may be linked to betel nut chewing, and, in the case of men, aggravated by heavy smoking.

Injections are preferred to oral medication, and patients frequently do not finish a course of tablets. To ensure correct compliance with a prescription, it is important to explain the likely side effects of a particular medicine.

Some patients expect home visits from their general practitioners for all ailments and are prepared to pay for them if necessary. Because of com-munication problems, surgery and hospital appointments are often missed. Women are particularly concerned not to be examined by a male doctor, and often fail to attend urology and gynaecology appointments if they cannot find an English speaking woman to attend with them. When visiting a doctor, husbands often prefer to accompany their wives, or for them to be escorted by a close relative or family friend.

Many Bangladeshis suffer from depression and anxiety as a result of poor housing conditions, unemployment, culture shock and racial harassment. Women are more prone to depression because of their social isolation.

Menstruation is seen as a healthy sign of fertility, and many Bangladeshi women worry about light periods, which can be interpreted by some to mean that something is wrong. Although family planning is now accepted, there is still a tendency to blame infertility on the woman, which can lead to divorce.

Further reading

Henley, A. (1982) *Caring for Muslims and their families: religious aspects of care*. Asians in Britain Series. National Extension College/DHSS/King's Fund Centre. National Extension College, Cambridge.

McAvoy, B.R. & Donaldson, L.J. (1990) *Health Care for Asians*. Oxford University Press, Oxford.

 National contacts _____

Dr Haroun Rashid
Albion Health Centre
Whitechapel Road
London E1 1BU
Tel: 0171 247 1730

Jahanara Loqueman, Shamsu Alam
or Rahima Hussain
Tower Hamlets Health Strategy Group
Oxford House
Derbyshire Street
London E2 6HG
Tel: 0171 729 9858

 Local contacts _____

✎ **Notes** _____

Chinese

The British Chinese community is concentrated in the West End of London, in Ealing, and in the London borough of Tower Hamlets. There is also a sizeable Chinese population in Manchester. The majority (over 75 per cent) of Chinese in Britain originate from Hong Kong. A smaller number of Chinese come from Singapore and Malaysia, in many cases to study. The remainder migrated from Vietnam, Taiwan and mainland China. Chinese people from Vietnam came as refugees ('boat people'), mostly after 1978.

The main phase of immigration from Hong Kong came in the 1950s and 1960s, partly in response to the collapse of traditional agriculture there, and because of the boom in the Chinese restaurant trade in Britain. About one third of the community are *Hakka* from rural areas of the colony who originally migrated to Hong Kong from North East China.

Immigration from Hong Kong may increase after the colony reverts to Chinese rule in 1997, although most Hong Kong residents wishing to emigrate have already made arrangements to live in Australia, Canada, USA and Singapore.

Languages

Most people from Hong Kong speak *Cantonese* as their first language, although *Hakka* or *Mandarin* may be the mother tongue for some. Most Singaporean and Malaysian Chinese speak *Hokien*, *Mandarin* or *Cantonese* as their first language. Taiwanese speak *Hokien*, *Taiwanese* or *Mandarin*, while most Vietnamese speak *Cantonese* and *Vietnamese*. All dialects are written in the Chinese script.

Many elderly members of the community do not speak, read or write English.

Naming systems and titles

The family name comes first, followed by a one- or two-part personal name, e.g. Cheung Chi Lam. A person's family of origin is of great significance; hence women traditionally preserve their maiden names. Many people have reversed their names, so that these correspond to the British naming pattern.

Health professionals should check which is the family name. Chinese Christians have Christian personal names, e.g. John Cheung.

Religion

Rather than subscribing to a single faith, many Chinese in Britain tend to be influenced by a variety of religions, principally Taoism, Confucianism and Buddhism. There is also a sizeable minority of Christians (mainly Roman Catholic, Protestant or Baptist), although these too are influenced by Taoist and Confucian beliefs. Most Christians from Hong Kong are Protestant.

The cardinal virtues of Confucianism are: *ee'yen* (benevolence), *yi* (duty, especially of a son towards his father), *li* (manners), *chih* (wisdom) and *hsin* (good faith and trustworthiness). Taoism is a philosophy that aims at achieving harmony with nature, and is particularly influential in Chinese attitudes to health (see below).

Also see 'Buddhism'.

Customs and relevant religious practices

Much emphasis is placed on family obligations, respect for the elderly, honesty and self-motivation. The worship of ancestors is perhaps the most salient religious feature of Chinese communities: funerals are thus very important. The Chinese believe that the soul has to be assisted on its way to heaven. Traditional religious practices include worship at temples and shrines, tending of shrines, offering food on feast days, and incense burning. Fortune telling and popular superstitions such as lucky and unlucky days are common.

Also see 'Buddhism'.

Festivals and holy days

The most important Chinese festivals are the New Year or Spring Festival, celebrated in February, the Dragon Boat festival in mid-summer and the Autumn festival in late August or September. Dates vary, as they are based on the lunar calendar.

Diet

There are few dietary taboos, although there is a strong preference for Chinese cuisine. Food is a very important element of Chinese culture, not only for social reasons but because of its effect on physical and mental well-being.

Food must, in theory at least, be balanced to achieve the harmony of *yin* and *yang* upon which the stability of life in general depends. Rice as the staple diet is regarded as an essential, almost holy, source of energy and nourishment. Chopsticks are used in preference to cutlery as eating utensils.

Birth

Great importance is attached to ante- and post-natal care within the Chinese communities. Women are urged to keep warm and avoid strenuous activity during pregnancy and following childbirth, and to protect their health and that of the infant at this vulnerable stage. Some women avoid cold drinks and do not wash their hair for several days after giving birth.

Death rites

Some families wrap the body in a special white shroud made from coarse material. Generally speaking, however, the deceased is buried in his or her best clothes. Some elderly people keep their own burial gowns in case their younger relatives will not know how to dress them after their death. Post mortems are not prohibited but are considered undesirable and distressing.

Medical restrictions

There are no official objections to blood transfusions or organ transplants. Some people worry about medical tests, in case they are weakened if too much blood is drawn off for samples.

Specific health issues

Among the older generation, traditional Chinese medicine, including acupuncture, is preferred to the conventional medical treatment available in Britain. Chinese pharmacies, selling a variety of herbs and roots, and acupuncture centres can be found in major 'chinatowns' in Britain. Chinese medical care is based on achieving a physical and mental state of balance within the body (*yin* and *yang*). Herbal teas, tonics and soups are recommended during convalescence.

NHS administrative procedures are often confusing for Hong Kong Chinese, because they are unfamiliar with a state health care system. For example, people may not be aware that they must register with a new doctor if they change address, or know how to get an appointment with a specialist after visiting their general practitioner. Women prefer to be examined by a female doctor. Among the elderly, poor English is a major obstacle to obtaining adequate health care.

Around 20 per cent of ethnic Chinese are thought to be hepatitis B carriers.

The incidence of naso-pharyngeal, oesophageal and stomach cancer in China is high. There are indications that these cancers also affect the Chinese in Britain.

Glucose-6-phosphate dehydrogenate (G6PD) deficiency is a comon disorder in South Chinese people. It also occurs in Thais, Filippinos and Mediterraneans. It is a sex-linked genetic disorder which causes haemolytic anaemia provoked by eating broad beans and the use of certain drugs, e.g. sulphonamides and anti-malarials. It may also cause neonatal jaundice in affected babies. Leaflets on G6PD deficiency can be obtained from The Centre for Inherited Blood Disorders, Abercronly Health Centre, Grove Street, Liverpool L7 7HG.

Heavy smoking is common, particularly among men.

Further reading

Li, Pui-Ling (1992) Health Needs of the Chinese Population. In: *The Politics of Race and Health* (ed. W.I.U. Ahmad). Race Relations Research Unit, Bradford University, Bradford.

Fong, C.L. (1995) Chinese health behaviour: breaking barriers to better understanding. *Health Trends*, **26**, 14–15.

☎ National contacts

Chinese Community Centre
44 Gerrard Street
London W1V 7LP
Tel: 0171 439 3822

Chinese Community Information Centre
146 Bromsgrove Street
Birmingham B5 6RG
Tel: 0121 622 3003/4039

Chinese Health Information Centre
1st Floor
39 George Street
Manchester M1 4HQ
Tel: 0161 228 0138

London Chinese Health Resource Centre
Queen's House
1 Leicester Place
Leicester Square
London WC2H 7BP
Tel: 0171 287 0904

Ms Luk Lin Tan
Camden Chinese Community Centre
173 Arlington Road
London NW1 7EY
Tel: 0171 267 3019

 Local contacts

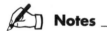 **Notes**

Cypriots - Greek

Some Greek Cypriots migrated to Britain before the Second World War, but the majority came here between 1954 and 1962. With the conflict in Cyprus in 1974 and the subsequent occupation of Northern Cyprus by Turkey, about 10 000 Greeks came to Britain as refugees. The Greek Cypriot community is mainly settled in North London, notably in Haringay. There are also significant communities in the South London district of Camberwell, and in Camden Town, where the original community was based. The Greek population in Britain is traditionally employed in small businesses, notably the leather and clothing industries. Many Greek Cypriots run small family businesses such as cafes, groceries, hairdressing and tailor shops. The community places much emphasis on the family and the community, and maintains a strong sense of ethnic identity.

Languages

Greek is often the only language spoken by the older generation. Younger members of the community are usually bilingual in English and Greek. The Greek spoken in Cyprus differs from mainland Greek in both spoken and written forms, much as British English differs from American English. A number of older people, especially women, are illiterate in Greek and have no knowledge of English.

Naming systems and titles

Surnames were often confused in the past because of administrative carelessness in Cyprus. The spelling of surnames was not standardised, leading to variations on individual names, e.g. Stylianou/Stylis. Matters were further complicated when some people decided to drop their family name and use their father's or grandfather's personal name as a surname. Some women use their husband's personal name as a surname; this applies particularly to the older generation.

Religion

Most Greeks are Christian – mainly Greek Orthodox – but there is a minority of Maronites and Jehovah's Witnesses.

Customs and relevant religious practices

The Greek Orthodox Church is an important focus for the community, and forms a major component of Greek Cypriot ethnic identity. Weddings, baptisms and funerals are often marked by elaborate ceremonies. Church attendance is high. Devout older people avoid eating meat during Lent and for two weeks before and after the Assumption, or may abstain from milk and dairy products, as well as oil and fried foods and sweets.

Festivals and holy days

The main religious festivals are Easter, Christmas and the feast of the Assumption of the Virgin Mary on 15 August.

Family planning

There are no religious prohibitions against the use of contraceptives, but abortions are not permitted.

Medical restrictions

Jehovah's Witnesses are not allowed blood transfusions.

Specific health issues

Thalassaemia is prevalent in this group, so much so, that marriages conducted in Cyprus are conditional upon the production of a document certifying the couple's thalassaemia status. Alcohol consumption, particularly at social occasions and in clubs is high among men, although this is not perceived as a problem by the community as a whole.

Further reading

Anthias, F. (1992) *Ethnicity, Gender and Migration* (Cypriots in London). Avebury, Aldershot.

 National contacts _____

Archbishop Gregorios
Church of All Saints
Pratt Street
Camden Town
London NW1
Tel: 0171 485 2149

Cypriot Advisory Service
26 Crowndale Road
London NW1 1TT
Tel: 0171 388 7971

Cypriot Community Centre
Earlham Grove
Wood Green
London N22 5HJ
Tel: 0181 881 2329

Thalassaemia Society,
United Kingdom
107 Nightingale Lane
London N8 7QV
Tel: 0181 348 0437

Greek Cypriot Women's
Association
Health Centre
Denmark Road
Hornsey
London N8 0DZ
Tel: 0181 341 5026

 Local contacts _____

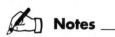 **Notes**

Cypriots – Turkish

The majority of the Turkish community in Britain comes from Cyprus, although a small number come from the Turkish mainland, often fleeing political persecution. (A clear distinction must be made between ethnic Turks and Kurds. Although the Kurds come mostly from Turkey, they constitute a separate ethnic and cultural group (see 'Kurds').)

The Turkish Cypriot community came to Britain in the aftermath of the inter-communal conflict between Greek and Turkish Cypriots in Cyprus during the 1960s and 1970s, and, in particular, after the Turkish invasion of Northern Cyprus in 1974 and the expulsion of about 20 000 ethnic Turks from the predominantly Greek South of the Island. This was carried out in reprisal for the displacement of 180 000 Greek Cypriots from the North.

Despite the animosity between Greek and Turkish Cypriots in Cyprus, inter-ethnic relations between the two communities in Britain are generally good.

The majority of Turkish Cypriots in Britain live in the London boroughs of Hackney, Haringay and Islington.

Languages

Older members of the community are often illiterate in their own language, and cannot speak English. But the younger generation now speak and write English as well as Turkish, and may be more fluent in English.

Naming systems and titles

Personal family names are used as they are in Britain. Many of them are Muslim in origin. Turkish uses the Latin alphabet, but some letters are pronounced differently and can cause confusion. For example, the surname Ciller is pronounced Chilair and an 'i' ending is pronounced 'uh'.

Religion

Islam is the religion practised by Turkish Cypriots.

Customs and relevant religious practices

See 'Islam'.

Specific health issues

Thalassaemia and pulpitis are a feature in this community.

Further reading

Anthias, F. (1992) *Ethnicity, Gender and Migration* (Cypriots in London). Avebury, Aldershot.

 National contacts _____

Cypriot Community Centre
Earlham Grove
Wood Green
London N22 5HJ
Tel: 0181 881 2329

The Cypriot Turkish Association
35 D'Arblay Street
London W1A 4YL
Tel: 0171 437 4940

Turkish Cypriot Cultural
Association
14a Graham Road
London E8 1DA
Tel: 0171 249 7410

Thalassaemia Society,
United Kingdom
107 Nightingale Lane
London N8 7QV
Tel: 0181 348 0437

 Local contacts _____

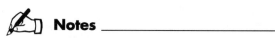

Notes

Eritreans

The Eritrean community in Britain consists mainly of refugees from the now independent region of Eritrea which lies along the Red Sea adjoining Ethiopia. Between 1962 and 1991 Eritreans were fighting for independence from Ethiopia and, as a result, thousands of Eritreans have been forced to take refuge in neighbouring countries such as Sudan and Kenya, but also in West European countries, including Britain. Independence was officially declared in May 1993, two years after the cessation of hostilities. In spite of this, few refugees have chosen to return.

Languages

The Eritreans speak mainly *Tigrinya* and Arabic. About 10 per cent of the community in Britain speak *Saho*, and approximately 20 per cent speak *Tigré*. Of these languages, only Arabic is written.

Naming systems and titles

Most people have a personal name followed by their father's name, and then by their grandfather's name. Most married women retain their maiden name.

Religion

Refugees from coastal and lowland Eritrea are usually Muslim, whereas highland Eritreans tend to be Eastern Orthodox Christians. The latter constitute approximately 60 per cent of the community in Britain.

Customs and relevant religious practices

In the case of Muslims, see 'Islam'.

Festivals and holy days

Most festivals are based on the religious calendar. See 'Islam' in the case of Muslims.

Social customs

Boys are normally circumcised before the age of two.

Female circumcision (or genital mutilation) by excision and infibulation is not common practice within the British Eritrean community, although it is still practised to some extent in Eritrea itself. The mildest form of the operation is sometimes referred to as *sunni*, and involves minor excision of the genital parts. The more severe version is known as *pharaonic* circumcision. This often results in chronic physical and mental suffering, and can give rise to severe infections due to the retention of urine and menstrual flow. Naturally, patients are often reluctant to report these conditions because they feel ashamed and embarrassed. Female circumcision has not yet been banned by the Eritrean government, although there is pressure to do so from progressive elements within the leadership.

Specific health issues

Like most refugees, Eritreans face problems of poor housing and unemployment, although the situation has improved in recent years. Many have suffered trauma and anxiety, and, in some cases, torture. One of the main barriers to proper health care provision remains language.

Further reading

No major references for this group are available.

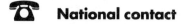 **National contact**

Tekle Berhe, Co-ordinator
Eritrean Community in the UK
266 Holloway Road
London N7 6NE
Tel: 0171 700 7995

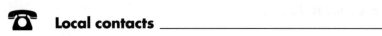 **Local contacts** _____

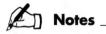 **Notes** _____

Ethiopians

The Ethiopian community in Britain came to this country in three different stages. The majority of the first group arrived before 1975 for education and business purposes. After the 1974 revolution many people were forced into exile. Some came to Britain as political refugees escaping from torture and persecution. This was followed by a wave of arrivals consisting mainly of young people in their teens seeking a better standard of life and refuge from compulsory military conscription. The most recent arrivals came after the collapse of the military regime in 1991, fleeing the resulting political and ethnic strife.

Languages

Ethiopia, traditionally known as Abyssinia, is characterised by remarkable cultural diversity and is home to a variety of ethnic groups speaking as many as 200 languages and dialects. The most prominent groups are the Amhara, the Oromo, the Gurages, Somalis and Tigré. Other important groups include the Afars and Issas from the desert region bordering the Red Sea. Amharic is the official language and is spoken and read by the majority of Ethiopians in Britain. (See separate entry for 'Eritreans'.)

Many older generation Ethiopians and recently-arrived exiles to not speak, read or write English, although Ethiopian community organisations have done much to alleviate this problem.

Naming systems and titles

Men are called *Ato* and women, *Wozeiro* or *Wozeirit*, equivalent to Mr, Mrs and Miss respectively. It used to be a common custom that senior people were addressed by additional titles such as *Ras*, *Dej-Azmatch*, *Fitawrari*, *Kegne-Azmatch*, *Gra-Azmatch*, *Balambaras* and *Bitweded*, as a mark of respect. Although this practice officially ended in 1974, with the fall of the old imperial rule, older people may still prefer to use these forms of address. Younger people are sometimes referred to as *Lij*. Surnames are not traditionally used. Christians use a personal name followed by a religious name, e.g. Haile-Mariam, Habte-Jesus or Saife-Michael, and finally by the father's or grandfather's name. Most of these names are based on the saint's day on which the child was born. Women usually retain their maiden names. Muslims adopt a similar sequence, but use Islamic names such as Muhammad Ali, Ali Mirah, Hussen and Abba Jiffar instead. Additional titles such as *Hajji* or *Sheikh* may be used according to the person's seniority in the community. There are also ceremonial titles such as *Demina, Garada, Ras Ali, Ali Mirah, Betweded*.

Religion

Both Islam and Christianity are practised in different parts of Ethiopia. Christians predominate in the highlands, while most Muslims come from the lowlands. The majority of Ethiopian Christians belong to the Ethiopian Orthodox Church which is a branch of the Eastern Orthodox Church. Most of the remainder are Pentecostalists.

Customs and relevant religious practices

For Muslims see 'Islam'.
Orthodox Christians place much emphasis on prayer, the worship of saints, and religious imagery, in particular icons and candles. The clergy have a very important role. Christmas is celebrated on 6 January (the Epiphany). Devout Christians traditionally fast for 55 days before Easter. Fasting in this sense means avoiding breakfast and animal products.

Pentecostalists believe in the necessity of experiencing the power and love of God, which is most vividly expressed in singing during services. Ecstatic experiences, divine healing and speaking in tongues are a feature of this religious denomination.

Birth

This is an especially celebrated occasion in the Ethiopian community and is accompanied by great festivities. Ante- and post-natal events are usually attended by family members and friends. Christian boys are baptised on the 40th day after birth. Both Christian and Muslim male infants are circumcised on the eighth day after birth.

Death rites

Burial is preferred. Funerals are a major social event. Traditionally, everyone in the community is expected to attend the service and visit the bereaved family during the three days following death. Mourning continues over a period of up to one year, and commemorations take place on the 40th day, in the sixth month after death, and on the anniversary of death for the next seven years.

Social customs

Female circumcision (or genital mutilation) by excision and infibulation is not common in Britain, although the operation is still prevalent among the Somali, Afar and Issa populations, and in some Tigrai and Amhara communities.

Specific health issues

The more recently arrived Ethiopian refugees face problems of disorientation, loss of identity, culture shock, uncertainty about immigration status, poor housing conditions and unemployment. There is often great anxiety about the fate of relatives left behind.

There is increasing concern among representatives of the Ethiopian community in Britain that many doctors fail to relate this high level of anxiety to the psycho-social and cultural background of these refugees. There is a strong need for psycho-social counselling as well as NHS medical treatment. Anecdotal evidence (see Further reading) exists for an increase in suicide rates (16 in the past year and a higher number of attempted suicides). There have also been unconfirmed reports of a higher incidence of schizophrenia among young Ethiopians, which will require further investigation.

Further reading

Karmi, G., Abdulrahim, D., Pierpoint, T. & McKeigue, P. (1992) *Suicide among Ethnic Minorities and Refugees in the UK*. The Health and Ethnicity Programme. NE and NW Thames Regional Health Authorities, London.

National contacts _____

Dr Girma Ejere
Ethiopian Community in Britain
66 Hampstead Road
London NW1 2NT
Tel: 0171 388 4944

Archbishop Yohannes Wolde
Gabriel
Ethiopian Orthodox Church
253b Ladbroke Grove
London W10 6HF
Tel: 0181 960 3848

Dr Zelalem Kebede
Ethiopian Health Support Project
10 Ebbsfleet Road
London NW2
Tel: 0181 450 1120

 Local contacts _____

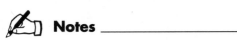 **Notes**

Ghanaians

Ghanaians in Britain originate from a wide variety of ethno-linguistic areas in Ghana, of which the Ashanti constitute the largest group.

Languages

Twi (*Ashanti, Akans*), *Dagbani, Ewe* (pronounced 'ayvay'), *Ga, Fanti, Hausa* and *Nzema*, as well as minor tribal languages and dialects, are all spoken.

Naming systems and titles

The traditional naming system is fairly complex. Ashantis name their children according to the day on which they were born, for example *Kwadjo* (masculine) and *Adjoa* (feminine), meaning Monday's child. Children are also given personal names and the name of a close relative or family friend with a good reputation. The father's name may be used as a surname, but this is not strictly necessary. The Ga-Adangbe people have special names for first-born children: *Tette* for boys and *Dede* for girls. Many family names have particular significance, denoting royal blood, as in the case of the Krobo Matekole, or indicating that the family is renowned for its high level of education, as in the case of the Ewe Acolatse.

Religion

People of Northern Ghana are likely to be Muslims or Catholics. Ghanaians from other parts may be Protestants, Methodists, Seventh Day Adventists or belong to a range of smaller Christian denominations.

Customs and relevant religious practices

See 'Islam' where relevant.

Diet

There are no specific dietary regulations. Some people may avoid certain foods, such as water yams or shellfish, on superstitious grounds because they believe them to be associated with evil influences in the family. The possibility of food allergies should not be ruled out.

Social customs

Customs depend very much on area of origin and degree of traditionalism. Circumcision is practised among Muslims and non-Muslims, although in the latter it is more a matter of custom rather than religious duty. Boys must be circumcised within seven days of birth; boys from the Ashanti or Akan aristocracy are exempt, but even this is not universally accepted nowadays. Female circumcision (excision and infibulation) is widespread, as it is throughout Sub-Saharan Africa (see 'Somalis').

Specific health issues

Sickle cell anaemia is a feature in this community.

Some older Ghanaians have little confidence in British conventional medicine and health practices and prefer self-diagnosis and self-medication for certain ailments. They have found that many medicines available over the counter in Ghana are not so easily obtainable in Britain. There is a preference for medication by injection, and many Ghanaians ask to be seen by a specialist immediately.

Further reading

No major references for this group are available.

☎ National contacts

Ghana Refugee Welfare Group
5 Westminster Bridge Road
London SE1 7XW
Tel: 0171 620 1430

Ghana Welfare Association
547–51 High Road
Leytonstone
London E11 4BP
Tel: 0181 558 9311

Sickle Cell Society
54 Station Road
Harlesden
London NW10 4UX
Tel: 0181 961 7795

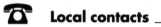 **Local contacts** _____

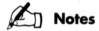 **Notes** _____

Gujaratis

Gujaratis constitute the largest group of South Asians in Britain. The majority came to Britain from Gujarat via East Africa (mainly Kenya and Uganda). A smaller proportion came directly from the state of Gujarat, which lies to the north of Bombay in India, and from the smaller region of Kutch close to the Pakistani border. Gujarati traders and railway workers settled in East Africa towards the end of the 19th century and, under British rule, Gujaratis became prominent in the East African business community. A large number of Ugandan Gujaratis were expelled by Idi Amin in 1972, and the majority fled to Britain.

Languages

Gujarati is the mother tongue of those members of the community born outside Britain. Some people speak Kutch, a dialect of Gujarati, and everyone speaks or understands some Hindi, as this is the *lingua franca* of Northern India. Both Gujarati and Hindi are written using different forms of the Devangri script. Many Gujarati women, especially those from lower social strata in rural areas of the subcontinent, are illiterate in their own language, and because they do not traditionally work outside the home, their English is often poor.

Naming systems and titles

Names consist of a first name, a middle name, and a family or sub-caste name, e.g. Chopra or Patel. The first and middle names are usually written as one name, e.g. Vijaykumar (Vijay plus Kumar). It is the custom for Gujarati men and unmarried women to use their fathers' names as their middle names. Married women adopt their husband's name.

Traditional forms of address use first and second names only. Title and family name, or title and full name are acceptable in Britain, e.g. Mr Patel or Mr Vijaykumar Patel. A small number of people have dropped their family name because of their objections to the caste system, and use their middle name as a surname.

Religion

The majority of Gujaratis are Hindus. A small number belong to the Jain sect which bears some resemblance to Buddhism with an emphasis on non-violence and respect for all living beings (*ahimsa*: meaning 'no killing'), as even the most insignificant insect is believed to have a soul. Jains also practise meditation, and are strict vegetarians.

There are small groups of Gujarati Muslims, Christians and Buddhists.

Specific health issues

Mortality from coronary heart disease is over 30 per cent higher than the national average.

The use of the eye cosmetic, *surma*, caused concern among health professionals during the 1980s, because it contained lead which could be absorbed through the eye. A prominent health education campaign launched since then has been successful in reducing the use of *surma*. A non-toxic alternative based on ash, known as *kajal*, is available.

As is the case in most South Asian groups, lactose intolerance (difficulty in digesting milk products) is said to exist in over 50 per cent of Gujaratis.

Further reading

Henley, A. (1983) *Caring for Hindus and their families: religious aspects of care.* Asians in Britain Series. National Extension College/DHSS/King's Fund Centre. National Extension College, Cambridge.

McAvoy, B. & Donaldson, L. (1990) *Health Care for Asians.* Oxford University Press, Oxford.

McKeigue, P. & Sevak, L. (1991) *Coronary Heart Disease in South Asian Communities. A Manual for Health Promotion.* Health Education Authority, London.

☎ National contacts

Gujarat Welfare Association
141 Plashet Road
Newham
London E13 0RA
Tel: 0181 552 0525

Mr Ramanbhai Barber
Gujarat Hindu Association
51 Loughborough Road
Leicester
Tel: 0116 2668266

Mr Nemu Chandaria
Institute of Jainology
Unit 18, Silicon Business Centre
26 Wandsworth Road
Greenford
Middlesex UB6 7JZ
Tel: 0181 997 2300

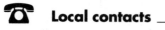 **Local contacts** _____

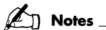 **Notes** _____

Iranians

Iranian migration to Britain began in earnest after the overthrow of the Shah in 1979 and the instalment of an Islamic Government in Iran under Ayatollah Khomeini. People came mainly to escape political persecution and safeguard their assets. In addition, many better-off Iranians who were used to a relatively liberal Western lifestyle in Iran under the Shah chose to live abroad, mainly in Europe and the United States. There followed a smaller wave of mainly young, middle class Iranians escaping military conscription during the war with Iraq (1980–88). Women unwilling to live by the strict religious code imposed on them in Iran, and a number of active political opponents of the Islamic regime, including members of ethnic minorities (see 'Kurds'), also came at the same time.

Cut off from their sources of income after the revolution (often as a result of appropriation by the state), many previously wealthy Iranians have seen their standard of living fall gradually over the years, whereas those who have managed to maintain strong links with their mother country have fared better.

The majority of Iranians in Britain live in West and North London.

Languages

The main language of Iran is *Farsi* (Persian), but about 15 million Iranians (approx 25 per cent of the total population) are ethnic Turks, who speak *Azeri* and other dialects of Turkish. Iran's Kurdish population, numbering 7 million, speaks *Kurdish*, and another 4 million or so people from South Eastern Iran have *Baluchi* as their mother-tongue. *Arabic* is widely spoken along the Gulf coast.

Naming systems and titles

Many Iranian surnames end in 'i', for example: Tehrani, Husseini, Javadi, Talei. Women retain their maiden names, but children adopt the father's surname. First names are usually religious in origin, but during the last Shah's reign (1943–79) old Persian names, such as Farhad, Parviz, Dariush and Khosrow, became fashionable among the better-off segments of the population.

Religion

The majority of Iranians (96 per cent) are Muslims, and of these 80 per cent belong to the *Shi'i* sect; the remainder, mostly Iranian Kurds, are *Sunni* Muslims. Other minority religious groups include Christians (Armenians, Nestorians, Protestants), Zoroastrians, Bahais and Jews.

Customs and relevant religious practices

See 'Islam'.

Shi'i Muslims have gained a reputation in the West for religious fanaticism in recent years. This is a result of the activities of the fundamentalist movement, which began in the 1970s and was enhanced by the rise to power of Ayatollah Khomeini in Iran. However, day-to-day practices do not differ significantly from those of *Sunni* Muslims. Many of those who settled in the West in the wake of the Iranian revolution follow the secular values promoted by the late Shah.

Fasting during the holy month of Ramadan is called *ruzeh* in Farsi.

Festivals and holy days

See 'Islam'.

The main religious event of the year for *Shi'i* Muslims is *Ashura*, commemorating the martyrdom of Hussein, on the 10th of *Moharram* (the first and holiest month of the Muslim calendar). *Nuruz*, the Persian new year, is celebrated on the spring equinox (around 21 March), and this is followed by the spring festival, *Sizdah-be-dar*, 13 days later. Other minor feasts include *Chahar Shambeh Souri*, the 'fire festival', of Zoroastrian origin, held on the last Tuesday of the year, and *Yaldeh*, the winter solstice.

Diet

Iranian cuisine is based largely on rice and various types of stews or grilled meats. Fresh fruit, fresh herbs and natural yoghurt are important components of the Iranian diet.

For dietary restrictions, see 'Islam'.

Specific health issues

Many Iranian refugees suffer from the physical and psychological effects of persecution. Some have been subjected to torture, while others live in fear of repatriation and the activities of their own security services.

Further reading

No major references for this group are available.

 National contacts _____

Iranian Community Centre
266–8 Holloway Road
London N7 6NE
Tel: 0171 700 0341

Dr Naser Adibi
Iranian Association
Palingswick House
241 King Street
London W6 9LP
Tel: 0181 748 6682

 Local contacts _____

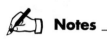 **Notes** _____

Japanese

The majority of Japanese people in Britain are temporary residents on three- to five-year contracts with Japanese companies operating in Britain. Unlike most other ethnic minority groups, the Japanese community has a high standard of living. As a result, health problems are not normally related to poor environmental or social conditions.

Languages

Although English is taught in all language schools, many Japanese are reluctant to speak it, and experience difficulty in comprehending spoken English.

Naming systems and titles

The personal name is followed by the surname, as in the West. People prefer to be addressed formally, and using first names can cause offence.

Religion

Although heavily secularised in recent years, most Japanese in Britain are, at least nominally, either Buddhists or Shintoists. Shinto, which literally means 'the way of the gods', or *kami*, is a set of social practices rather than religious beliefs. State Shinto, which claimed the divinity of the Emperor, was disestablished after the Second World War. Shinto is still practised today in a much modified form.

Customs and relevant religious practices

See 'Buddhism' where appropriate.

Festivals and holy days

The main religious festivals are New Year, the Spring Festival and the feast of the lanterns (All Souls).

Diet

Japanese dishes usually include rice, which is a staple food in Japan. Raw fish, seaweed and raw eggs are often eaten. Clear fish and soya-based soups are also common. The traditional Japanese diet has a low meat content, soya bean protein being used instead. Many Western foods are not appreciated, particularly by older Japanese.

Medical restrictions

There are no restrictions based on religious objections; practices depend on personal beliefs.

Specific health issues

There is a raised incidence of gastric ulcer and cancer of the stomach, which has been associated with the consumption of large amounts of pickled foods.

Further reading

No major references for this group are available.

☎ National contact

Japan Information and Cultural Centre
Embassy of Japan
101–104 Piccadilly
London W1V 9FN
Tel: 0171 465 6500

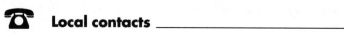 **Local contacts**

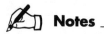 **Notes**

Kurds

The Kurdish national homeland, Kurdistan, extends across North Western Iran, North Eastern Iraq, much of Eastern Turkey, and parts of Syria, and the Caucasus. There is also a small Kurdish community in Lebanon. The Kurds have been unable to achieve their goal of self-determination, and Kurdish nationalism has led to harsh, often violent, counter-measures by the national governments concerned and a continuing regional conflict. As a result, many Kurds have sought refuge outside the region, especially in Western Europe.

Languages

The Kurdish language, spoken and written, is used by all Kurdish migrants irrespective of country of origin, although different dialects are used: *Kurmanji*, spoken in North Eastern Turkey and the former Soviet Union (written in the Latin and Cyrillic scripts respectively); *Sorani*, used by Kurds from Iraq (in the Arabic script); *Kirmanshahi*, *Leki* and *Gurani*, spoken in Iran; and *Zaza* spoken in the Dersim region of Eastern Turkey. Some Kurds coming from Turkey use Turkish, since their own language has been outlawed there for many years. Kurdish refugees are generally reluctant to speak in what they regard as the languages of their oppressors. Kurdish is, therefore, the preferred language for interpreting purposes.

Naming systems and titles

There is no specific naming system. In some cases the personal name is followed by the father's, then by the grandfather's name or by the name of a close relative, reflecting the traditions of a society that was, until recently, tribal. Married women tend to adopt their husband's family name. Some parents name their children after well-known Kurdish national figures.

Religion

The majority of Kurdish refugees in Britain are Muslims of the *Alevi* sect, which is closely related to *Shi'ism*, although the majority of Kurds in Kurdistan are *Sunni* Muslims.

Customs and relevant religious practices

See 'Islam'.

Festivals and holy days

The birth of the prophet (*Mawlid*) is a particularly important festival. For Iranian Kurds, the most popular non-religious festival is *Nowruz* on 21 March, which marks the New Year and the first day of spring.

Social customs

Many Kurds resident in Britain have adopted certain aspects of Western lifestyle, such as European dress and a more liberal attitude to the mixing of the sexes. Nevertheless, Islamic cultural norms still predominate, and women prefer to be examined by female medical staff.

Specific health issues

The main reasons for fleeing to Britain were to escape military service, persecution, and, in many cases, physical torture. In addition, many Iraqi Kurds suffered from severe repression, including enforced internal migration, and the use of chemical weapons against them. As a result, many Kurds are prone to stress, anxiety and depression.

Further reading

No major references for this group are available.

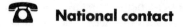 **National contact**

Kurdish Cultural Centre
14 Stannary Street
London SE11 4AA
Tel: 0171 735 0918

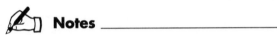 **Local contacts** _____

✍ **Notes** _____

Nigerians

Most Nigerians resident in Britain come from the Yoruba-speaking South and West, and from the Ibo-speaking Eastern areas of Nigeria. The majority come here to study.

Languages

Yoruba, Ibo and Hausa are all spoken. Yoruba is widely understood, as it is the language of the capital, Lagos, as is English. Hausa is the usual language of business in West Africa, and is spoken in the North of Nigeria.

Naming systems and titles

In addition to personal names, people may have others indicating the day and place of their birth and may also have been given the name of a close relative or family friend. Some names commemorate an important event. A boy, for example, may be given the name 'Ade' if a tribal chief is crowned on the day of his birth.

Religion

Islam and various Christian denominations, including Roman Catholic, Anglican, Protestant, the Church of Christ, Seventh Day Adventists and other sects are all represented. Most of the Muslims come from the Hausa and Yoruba areas. The ratio of Muslims to Christians among the Nigerian community in Britain is approximately 50:50.

Specific health issues

Sickle cell disease is a feature in this community.

Female circumcision (excision and infibulation) is widely practised in many parts of West Africa, including Nigeria. The custom transcends religious and cultural boundaries, although individual tribes, such as the Fulani and the

Nupes disapprove of the custom. The milder form of the operation is sometimes referred to as *sunni* and involves minor excision of the genital parts. The more severe version, known as *pharaonic* circumcision, involves the removal of the inner labia and stitching of the entrance to the vagina to leave only a small hole. The latter is rare in Nigeria.

Further reading

No major references for this group are available.

 National contacts _____

African Welfare and Immigration
Advisory Centre
200 The Grove
Stratford
London E15 1LS
Tel: 0181 519 6935

Sickle Cell Society
54 Station Road
Harlesden
London NW10 4UX
Tel: 0181 961 7795

 Local contacts _____

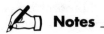 **Notes**

Punjabis – Pakistanis

The majority of Pakistanis are ethnic Punjabis, from the province of Punjab, in North East Pakistan. A smaller number come from the cities of Karachi and Islamabad, from the Mirpur district in Pakistani Kashmir and from the North-West Frontier province along the Afghan border. Some Punjabi Pakistanis migrated from East Africa, where their families had settled at the end of the 19th century. Punjabis in Britain can be divided into several groups. Those coming from the Pakistani state of Punjab are Muslim, while those from the Indian province of the same name are usually Hindus or Sikhs. After the partition of the Indian subcontinent into India and Pakistan in 1947, the Punjab region was divided between the two countries along the new frontier. The partition was the cause of extensive inter-ethnic violence at the time.

Languages

Punjabi is spoken and written by people from the Punjab and from Mirpur, and by many East African Asians. Pashtu is spoken by the Pathans (Afs) from the North-West Frontier Province, bordering Afghanistan. People from the cities and the more educated migrants speak and read Urdu, which is the national language, written in the Arabic script. There are also regional dialects used by some Pakistanis in Britain, such as Sindhi, Baluchi and Kashmiri. Illiteracy is not uncommon in the Pakistani community, particularly among women. Many of those from rural areas and from lower social strata cannot read or write their own language. In addition, many older Pakistani women in Britain cannot speak, read or write English, as they usually do not work outside the home, and therefore have little contact with people other than their own families.

Naming systems and titles

Pakistani men have two or three names, of which at least one has religious significance, e.g. Ali Rahman, Gulam Khan, Mohammad Khalid Qureishi. Pakistani women usually have two names, such as Amina Begum, Fatma Khatoon. The first two names are used together when addressing someone. Using just one name alone is not acceptable.

Asian Muslims do not traditionally adopt a family surname. Therefore, every family member will have a different last name, which can cause confusion among those recording patient particulars. Children born in Britain usually adopt their father's last name. Women retain their own name after marriage.

Religion

Islam is the religion of this group.

Customs and relevant religious practices

See 'Islam'.

Fasting is known as *roza* in Urdu. Traditional dress (*shalwar kameez*) for women consists of a long tunic with long or half sleeves worn with very loose trousers. Clothes are cut wide for comfort and modesty. A long scarf (*chuni, dupatta*) is also worn, and can be used to cover the head. The *shalwar kameez* is also worn as bedtime clothing.

Festivals and holy days

See 'Islam'.

Diet

Bread (*chapatis*) and meat, especially beef and lamb, are staple foods. Because they are Muslim, Pakistanis do not eat pork, and only eat meat that is *halal* (see 'Islam'). The consumption of alcohol is forbidden, as with other Muslims.

Specific health issues

As in all the groups from the Indian sub-continent, there is a significant risk of coronary heart disease and diabetes in this group.

There is also a high rate of perinatal mortality – the highest for any ethnic group in Britain. This has been linked to congenital malformations which may be related to the high frequency of consanguineous (first cousin) marriage in this group. Thalassaemia is also common because of this.

Traditional *unani* medicine is used by some people, who also consult *hakims* (traditional healers). Some of the traditional remedies used contain toxic metals and may be a health hazard.

In common with other South Asians, over half the Punjabi population are thought to be lactose intolerant, i.e. cannot digest milk products.

Further reading

Balarajan, R. & Botting, B. (1989) Perinatal mortality in England and Wales: variation by mother's country of birth (1982–5). *Health Trends*, **21**, 79–84.

Henley, A. (1982) *Caring for Muslims and their families: religious aspects of care*. Asians in Britain Series. National Extension College/DHSS/ King's Fund Centre. National Extension College, Cambridge.

McAvoy, B. & Donaldson, L. (1990) *Health Care for Asians*. Oxford University Press, Oxford.

☎ National contacts

Mohamed Azam
Pakistan Society
28 Saint Thomas Street South
Coppice
Oldham
Lancashire OL8 1SG

*Pakistani Women's Welfare
Association*
20 Blackstock Road
London N4 2DW
Tel: 0171 226 4427

Pakistani Welfare Association
1a Station Road
London SE25 5AH
Tel: 0181 653 6505

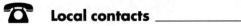 **Local contacts** _____

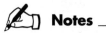 **Notes** _____

Somalis

There has been a small Somali community in Britain, predominantly in East London, Sheffield and Cardiff since the end of the 19th century. The earliest immigrants were merchant seamen. Their families stayed behind in Somalia and they went back to visit them periodically. Between 1965 and 1975, many of these families came to settle in Britain permanently.

Since the outbreak of civil war in Somalia in 1988, a large proportion of the population of the north of the country (the independent Republic of Somaliland since 1993) has been displaced. Many fled to neighbouring Ethiopia and Kenya, and a few to Western Europe. After the January 1991 fall of General Siyad Barré, a civil war also broke out in Southern Somalia, which resulted in hundreds of thousands of people fleeing to Ethiopia, Kenya, Yemen and the West.

Most of the Somalis in Britain are settled in the East London boroughs of Tower Hamlets and Hackney. There is also a growing community in Ealing.

Languages

Somali is the official medium of communication in Somalia. Arabic is often learned as a second language, as are English and Italian (Italy having been the former colonial power). The Somali language was not written until 1972, when it was agreed to use the Latin alphabet. Many newly arrived refugees have a very limited knowledge of English which hinders their integration into the local community. A high proportion of older generation Somalis are not literate in any language.

Naming systems and titles

One or two personal names are adopted usually followed by the father's or grandfather's name. Family names are not used as they are in the West, i.e. may not be shared by members of the same family. Names may be prefixed by a religious title such as 'Aw', 'Sheikh' and 'Hajji' which means that the person has memorised the Qur'an (Koran).

Religion

Islam is the religion of the Somalis.

Customs and relevant religious practices

See 'Islam'.

Social customs

Use of the mild stimulant known as *qat* is very common among Somali men. The drug comes in the form of leaves, and is chewed at social gatherings, often for hours.

Specific health issues

Somali refugees face numerous problems, ranging from poor understanding of the social security system to sub-standard housing conditions, unemployment and culture shock. Many skilled and once prosperous Somalis have seen their living standards decline drastically. Somali refugees are often unfamiliar with such procedures as enrolling their children at school or registering with a local general practitioner. Language problems aggravate all these problems.

In addition to the anxieties caused by resettlement and readjustment, many Somalis suffer from depression and trauma as a result of their experiences of civil war and torture in Somalia. Some have lost all their relatives while others fear for the safety of those left behind.

Female circumcision by excision and infibulation is commonly carried out on Somali women, and girls as young as five may be operated on. Although circumcision is officially banned in Somalia, it is firmly entrenched in traditional culture and is still widely practised. Problems have arisen in this country because members of the Somali community want to have the operation carried out, although it is illegal. The mildest form of the operation is sometimes referred to as *sunni* and involves minor excision of the genital parts. The more severe version, known as *pharaonic* circumcision, involves the removal of the inner labia and stitching of the entrance to the vagina to leave only a small hole. This often results in chronic physical and mental suffering, and can give rise to severe infections, due to the retention of urine and menstrual flow. Naturally, patients are often reluctant to report these conditions because they feel ashamed and embarrassed.

Further reading

No major references for this group are available.

 National contacts _____

Saadia Ahmed
Somali Interpreting Project
Oxford House
Derbyshire Street
London E2 6HG
Tel: 0171 739 9001

Mohamud Ahmed
Tower Hamlets Health Strategy Group
Oxford House
Derbyshire Street
London E2 6HG
Tel: 0171 729 9858

Somali Mental Health Council Project Ltd
5 Westminster Bridge Road
London SE1 7XW
Tel: 0171 620 4589

 Local contacts _____

Notes

Sudanese

Sudan is strongly divided along ethnic lines: the Northern two-thirds of the country is Muslim and Arabic speaking (see also 'Arabs'), while the South is home to many different Christian and Animist tribal groups. The number of refugees increased sharply following the *coup d'etat* by a fundamentalist Muslim dictatorship in 1989. Many refugees are non-Muslims from the South of Sudan, who were engaged in a struggle with the military regime. Others are people who were facing persecution because of their beliefs, such as Christians, liberals, educated professionals, civil rights activists, priests, members of the Coptic Church and political opponents of the regime.

About half the Sudanese population in Britain are refugees. The remainder are short-term visitors, such as students and businessmen. A relatively large proportion of the community are educated professionals, notably doctors.

Most members of the Sudanese community live in London and Manchester. About 1000 Sudanese Copts live in Brighton.

Languages

Arabic is the first language of about half the population, and the language of administration and education. A variety of different central African languages are spoken in the south of the country.

Naming systems and titles

Surnames are not used, except for official purposes. Wives retain their maiden names.

Religion

Most Arabic-speakers are *Sunni* Muslims, who adhere to indigenous Sufi orders known as *tariqas*. These preach a mystical and tolerant form of Islam. Christianity and various Animist and pagan religions predominate in the South. A small minority of people from the North of Sudan belong to the Coptic Church, an ancient branch of Orthodox Christianity that evolved in neighbouring Egypt.

Customs and relevant religious practices

See 'Islam'.

Social customs

Weddings, funerals and births are attended by large numbers of relatives and friends, and hospital patients may receive a steady stream of visitors. Guests are highly honoured. Among many Muslim Sudanese women, it is customary to hold parties, where they perform a rhythmic dance, often leading to an ecstatic trance-like state. The purpose of these occasions is to provide an opportunity for women to enjoy themselves, and release stress due to the strict regulations imposed by custom on female behaviour.

Specific health issues

Female circumcision (excision and infibulation) is widespread amongst Muslim women in Sudan, although strictly speaking it is not a religious practice. Female circumcision often results in chronic physical and mental suffering, and in its most severe form (see under 'Somalis') can give rise to severe infections, due to the retention of urine and menstrual flow. Naturally, patients are often reluctant to report these conditions because they feel ashamed and embarrassed. Illegal circumcisions are reportedly carried out privately in Britain, often by non-medical staff.

There is an increased prevalence of respiratory tract infections and asthma, perhaps brought on by the cold, damp weather conditions in Britain.

Language is a major barrier to health care, particularly for women, who live mainly within the family circle and with Sudanese friends, and therefore have little opportunity for speaking English.

Further reading

No major references for this group are available.

National contacts _____

Dr Ahmed Gasim
Sudanese Doctors Union
31 St Edward Gardens
Eggbuckland
Plymouth PL6 5PB
Tel: 01752 778489

Dr Nadia (Fridays only)
Sudanese Community Information Centre
14 Newton Road
London W2
Tel: 0171 229 4338

Sudanese Coptic Association
23 Embassy Court
Kings Road
Brighton BN1 2PX
Tel: 01273 328833

 Local contacts _____

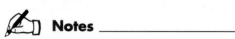 **Notes**

Tamils

The Tamil community in Britain comes mainly from Sri Lanka and from the southern Indian state of Tamil Nadu. A minority come from Malaysia and Singapore.

Since the outbreak of inter-ethnic violence in Sri Lanka between the Tamil (mainly Hindu) minority and the Sinhalese (Buddhist) majority in the mid-1980s, many Tamils have sought refuge in Britain.

Languages

Tamil is spoken.

Naming systems and titles

In the case of Hindus, the naming system is as follows: father's name plus personal name for men and personal name plus father's name for women. Christian Tamils use family names for surnames, as in Europe.

Religion

About 80 per cent of the Tamil community in Britain are Hindus, 15 per cent are Christian, and the remainder are Muslim.

Customs and relevant religious practices

See 'Hinduism' or 'Islam' as appropriate.

Diet

Hindus are vegetarian.

Specific health issues

As in other South Asian ethnic groups in Britain, there is a raised incidence of coronary heart disease. Lactose intolerance (inability to digest milk products) is also prevalent in this community.

Tamil refugees have a history of persecution and, in some cases, physical torture. Many are anxious about families left behind and many also fear forcible repatriation, and therefore live in a constant state of insecurity. Many Tamils suffer from the effects of anxiety and trauma.

Further reading

No major references for this group are available.

 National contacts _____

Dr T. Moorthy
Tamil Refugee Action Group
335 Grays Inn Road
London WC1X 8PX
Tel: 0171 833 2020

Medical Institute of Tamils
Tamil House
720 Romford Road
London E12 6BT
Tel: 0181 553 2692

 Local contacts _____

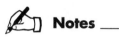 **Notes**

Traveller-Gypsies

Traveller-Gypsies are one of the oldest ethnic minorities in Britain, dating back to the 16th century, and possibly earlier. The Traveller population can roughly be divided into two groups: Irish/Scottish Travellers (Tinkers), who are mainly of indigenous origin; and English/Welsh Travellers, who are thought to descend, originally, from a group of people who began to migrate westwards from the Indian sub-continent in the 11th century AD. However, the two groups have mixed over the centuries and now share a similar ethnic identity, based on a nomadic existence. Because Traveller-Gypsies have only recently been recognised as a separate ethnic group, discrimination against them was not an offence under the Race Relations Act until 1989.

It is important to note that Traveller-Gypsies are nomadic by tradition, and are not to be confused with New Age Travellers, who are essentially settled people who have chosen to opt out of mainstream society in recent years.

For practical purposes, Traveller-Gypsies can be defined as follows:

'Nomadic families who by reason of their lifestyle habitually travel to sell the products of their self-employment and to pick up casual or seasonal work, and whose only or main residence is a caravan or tent for which they have no permanent site.'

(Wibberley 1986)

It is estimated that there are at least 50 000 Traveller-Gypsies in Britain, and a similar number of settled Gypsies who share Traveller cultural values to a certain extent but are not covered by the above definition. Traveller-Gypsies have always been the object of prejudice by the settled community, and this has made it difficult for them to find suitable land for camping, whether private or public. The Traveller community now faces the additional threat of a change to the Caravan Site Act 1968, which obliged local authorities to provide suitable sites for Travellers. If passed, the new Act will remove this statutory obligation and make parking on an unauthorised site a criminal offence.

Languages

English and Romanes (Romany) which varies according to the area. Romanes is heavily anglicised as a result of centuries of interaction with English-speakers, but also contains many loan-words from cultures the group came into contact with prior to arrival in Britain. In addition to English, non-Romany Travellers, who are descended from indigenous Irish and British nomads, speak Shelta, or, in the case of Scottish Travellers, Gammer. Many Traveller-Gypsies are illiterate.

Naming systems and titles

Children do not automatically adopt their father's surname, and wives often choose to keep their own surnames, or adopt those of other relatives. Names tend to reflect the region of origin. Thus, Traveller-Gypsies from Ireland, Scotland and Wales adopt names typical of those countries. Common surnames among English Gypsies include names such as Smith, Wood, Wilson, Lee and Young. Travellers tend to have more than one name, for use in different circumstances. Sometimes, an entirely new name may be adopted, replacing the name given at birth.

Religion

Traveller-Gypsies from Ireland are Catholic. The others are mostly Protestant.

Diet

Many Travellers will not eat hospital food, or any food prepared out of their sight, for fear that it may be 'unclean'. Tinned food is often more acceptable.

Birth

There is universal preference for hospital births. Childbirth is seen as a *mochadi* ('polluting') life event, and therefore best left to the assistance of outsiders. The mother and baby are also regarded as *mochadi* for some time after birth, as are the sheets, bed and any other items closely associated with the event. There is a preference for bottle-feeding among Traveller mothers.

Death rites

Death is a very important occasion. There is much outward expression of grief and funerals are heavily attended. The task of handling and preparing the body for burial is carried out by non-Gypsies. To avert misfortune, all possessions belonging to the deceased are normally destroyed or discarded.

Social customs

Concepts of health and hygiene differ considerably from those of settled people. There is an emphasis on 'inner purity' as opposed to 'public health'. This is reflected in Gypsy camps by the contrast between the concern for immaculate cleanliness and tidiness inside the home, and the relative disregard for environmental conditions surrounding the camp. Inner cleanliness for Gypsies also means avoiding things they regard as mochadi ('polluting'), which covers most things outside their community. This includes hospitals and surgeries, which are viewed as places of 'illness' and 'death' and hence to be avoided, except in emergencies. This 'inner' and 'outer' cleanliness concept underlies the strong Gypsy sense of 'us and them', which is constantly confirmed by prejudice and animosity towards the Traveller community from Gorgios (non-Gypsies). As a result, access to the community can be difficult.

Because female modesty is highly praised, contact with unrelated men is frowned upon, and women prefer to be examined by female medical staff.

Specific health issues

Access to primary health care is a major problem. The conventional appointment systems and the administrative procedures of hospitals and general practitioner surgeries are inappropriate for the majority of Travellers, who have no fixed address, and therefore no telephone or postal delivery. Illiteracy means Travellers are often unable to fill in forms or read prescriptions and appointment cards. There are reports of general practitioners not accepting Travellers as patients, and Travellers have also reported hostility towards them from staff at antenatal and child clinics. However, access has been improving slowly since the appointment of specialist outreach workers by some health authorities.

Because intermarriage is common, the risk of transmitting autosomal recessive disorders, such as phenylketonuria, is high. Uptake of immunisation is poor, and there have been reports of infection with polio, TB and tetanus. Accidents among children are frequent, often because of hazards present at Traveller encampment sites. In addition, children are exposed to lead and other pollutants because of the proximity of camps to busy roads. The general standard of health in this group is poorer than in the settled population as a whole. This is reflected in lower than average life expectancy, and a higher reported incidence of gastro-intestinal, respiratory tract and chronic skin infections, particularly among children.

Heavy cigarette smoking is common.

Further reading

Feder, G. (1989) Traveller-Gypsies and primary care. *Journal of the Royal College of General Practitioners*, **39**, 425.

Hawes, D. & Perez, B. (1995) *The Gypsy and the State*. School of Advanced Urban Studies, University of Bristol, Bristol.

Okely, J. (1983) *The Traveller-Gypsies*. Cambridge University Press, Cambridge.

Wibberley, G.A. (1986) *A Report on the Analysis of Responses to Consultation on the Operation of the Caravan Sites Act, 1968*. Department of the Environment, London.

 National contacts _____

Dr Gene Feder
*Department of General Practice
and Primary Care*
The Medical Colleges of
St Bartholomew's and the
Royal London Hospitals
Charterhouse Square
London EC1M 6BQ
Tel: 0171 982 6100

National Gypsy Council
Greengate Street
Oldham
Lancashire OL4 1DG
Tel: 0161 665 1924

*Advisory Committee for the
Education of Romany and other
Travellers*
Moot House
The Stow
Harlow
Essex CM20 3AG
Tel: 01279 418666

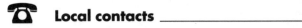 **Local contacts** _____

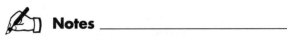 **Notes** _____

Vietnamese

Since 1975, and especially after 1978, many Vietnamese have fled their country for political and economic reasons. A substantial number have settled in Britain, many arriving via Hong Kong. Over 70 per cent of Vietnamese immigrants are ethnic Chinese, approximately 16 per cent ethnic Vietnamese and the remainder are Laotians or Kampucheans. Most refugees in this group come from the rural areas of former North Vietnam.

Languages

Most Vietnamese people speak both Vietnamese and Cantonese. Many refugees, however, come from relatively underdeveloped areas in northern Vietnam and cannot read or write either language. Knowledge of English is poor. Most refugees were given intensive language training on arrival, but men tended to receive more tuition than women, because women were more preoccupied with children and domestic affairs. Generally speaking, the standard of written and spoken English among first generation immigrants is low.

Naming systems and titles

A family name is used followed by a middle name then a first name. This is often reversed in Britain for administrative purposes.

Religion

Vietnamese religious life is centred around Buddhism, but is also influenced by the Chinese philosophies of Taoism and Confucianism. Many Vietnamese, however, have grown up in an atheist environment under the Communist Government.

Customs and relevant religious practices

See 'Buddhism'.

Festivals and holy days

Vietnamese celebrate the Lunar (Chinese) New Year. Another main occasion for celebration is the family festival which falls on the fifth day of the fifth month of the lunar calendar.

Diet

Some Vietnamese are vegetarians and others abstain from eating meat for ten days each month or during the whole month of July. This is a personal choice. Rice is the staple food.

Death rites

In Britain, cremation is the usual option taken. Some Vietnamese prefer to be embalmed.

Social customs

Obligations to family members and respect for the elderly are important features of this community. Ancestor worship is also a key cultural value, as are hospitality and self-reliance. It is regarded as a sign of respect to lower the eyes when speaking to a more senior person.

Specific health issues

Approximately 10–20 per cent of adults in South East Asia (Vietnam, Thailand, Laos, Kampuchea and Burma) are carriers of Hepatitis B.

Vietnamese children have an increased prevalence of dental caries.

Adaptation to life in Britain has been particularly difficult for the Vietnamese, because of wide cultural differences and an unfamiliar environment. Some Vietnamese still suffer psychological scars of stress experienced in refugee camps in Hong Kong and other parts of South East Asia.

Further reading

Bedi, R. & Elson, R.A. (1991) Dental caries and oral cleanliness of Asian and caucasian children aged 5 and 6 attending primary schools in Glasgow and Trafford, UK. *Community Dental Health*, **8**, 17–23.

National contacts _____

Derby Vietnamese Community
Association
91 Dairy House Road
Derby DE23 8HQ
Tel: 01332 291318

Vietnamese Refugee National
Council
25 Station Road
London SE25 5AH
Tel: 0181 771 8960

Vietnamese Refugee Project
115 Powis Street
London SE18 6JL
Tel: 0181 854 9907

The An Viet Foundation
12 Englefield Road
London N1 4LN
Tel: 0171 275 7521

 Local contacts _____

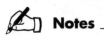 **Notes**

Bibliography

Health and ethnicity

Ahmad, W.I.U. (ed.) (1992) *The Politics of 'Race' and Health.* Race Relations Research Unit, University of Bradford, Bradford.

Balarajan, R. & Raleigh, V.S. (1993) *Ethnicity and Health.* Department of Health, London.

Chan, M. (1995) *Chinese Health in Britain – the Way Forward.* Leeds University Press, Leeds.

Collins, D., Tank, M. & Basith, A. (1993) *Customs of Minority Ethnic Religions.* Arena, Aldershot.

Cruickshank, J.K. & Beevers, D.G. (eds) (1989) *Ethnic Factors in Health and Disease.* Butterworth-Heinemann, Guildford.

Helman, C.G. (1990) *Culture, Health and Illness: an Introduction for Health Professionals.* Wright, London.

Her Majesty's Stationery Office (1991) *Ethnic Minorities.* Aspects of Britain Series. Her Majesty's Stationery Office, London.

Hopkins, A. & Bahl, V. (eds) (1993) *Access to Health Care for People from Black and Ethnic Minorities.* Royal College of Physicians, London.

Karmi, G. & McKeigue, P. (eds) (1993) *The Ethnic Health Bibliography.* NE and NW Thames Regional Health Authorities, London.

McAvoy, B.R. & Donaldson, L.J. (eds) (1990) *Health Care for Asians.* Oxford University Press, Oxford.

Smaje, C. (1995) *Health, Race and Ethnicity.* Share/King's Fund, London.

Minority ethnic groups

Anthias, F. (1992) *Ethnicity, Gender and Migration* (Cypriots in London). Avebury, Aldershot.

Bhachu, P. (1985) *Twice Migrant – A Study of the Sikh Community in Britain.* Tavistock, London.

Bhat, A., Carr-Hill, R. & Ohri, S. (1988) *Britain's Black Population.* Gower, London.

Booth, H. (1992) *The Migration Process in Britain and West Germany.* Avebury, Aldershot.

Castles, S. (1987) *Here for Good – Western Europe's new Ethnic Minorities*. Pluto Press, London.

Chandan, A. (1986) *Indians in Britain*. Oriental University Press, London.

Her Majesty's Stationery Office (1991) *Ethnic Minorities*. Aspects of Britain Series. Her Majesty's Stationery Office, London.

Rex, J. & Mason, D. (1986) (ESRC) *Theories of Race and Ethnic Relations*. Cambridge University Press, Cambridge.

Roosens, E. (1989) *Creating Ethnicity*. Anthropological Series. Sage, London.

Religion

Collins, D., Tank, M. & Basith, A. (1993) *Customs of Minority Ethnic Religions*. Arena Publications, Aldershot.

Henley, A. (1982) *Caring for Muslims and their families; Caring for Sikhs and their families; Caring for Hindus and their families*. Asians in Britain Series. National Extension College/DHSS/King's Fund Centre. National Extension College, Cambridge.

Weller, P. (1993) *Religions in the UK – A Multi-faith Directory*. University of Derby/Inter-faith Network for the UK, Derby.

Useful Addresses

This is not an exhaustive list of community organisations. Only the main ones have been included, as many groups are very small or operate for only a transient period. Central organisations should be contacted for the addresses of local branches. For refugee organisations, the Refugee Council should be contacted first. Telephone numbers have been included where they were made available.

Association of Black Social Workers and Allied Professions
The Eurolink Business Centre
Effra Road
London SW2 1BZ
Tel: 0171 738 5603

British Diabetic Association
10 Queen Anne Street
London W1M 0BD
Tel: 0171 323 1531

CARILA Latin American Welfare Group
5 Bradbury Street
London N16 8JN
Tel: 0171 275 8698

Commission for Racial Equality
Elliot House
10-12 Allington Street
London SW1E 5EH
Tel: 0171 828 7022

Ethnic Minority Resource Centre
5 Westminster Bridge Road
London SE1 7XW
Tel: 0171 928 0095

Institute of Race Relations
2–6 Leeke Street
London WC1X 9HS
Tel: 0171 837 0041

Joint Council for the Welfare of Immigrants
115 Old Street
London EC1V 9JR
Tel: 0171 251 8706

Leeds Black Communities AIDS Team
Ms Iris Berkeley, Coordinator
50 Call Lane
Leeds LS1 6DT
Tel: 0113 242 3100

Local Authority Race Relations Information Exchange (LARRIE)
38 Belgrave Square
London SW1X 8NZ
Tel: 0171 259 5464

London Black Women's Health Action Project
Community Centre
1 Cornwall Avenue
London E2 0HW
Tel: 0181 980 3503

London Interpreting Project (LIP)
20 Compton Terrace
London N1 2UN
Tel: 0171 359 6798

*Medical Foundation for the Care
of Victims of Torture*
96–8 Grafton Road
London NW5 3EJ
Tel: 0171 284 4321

Migrants' Resource Centre
24 Churton Street
London SW1V 2LP
Tel: 0171 834 2505

Migrant Support Unit
6–20 John's Mews
Holborn
London WC1 2XN
Tel: 0171 916 1646

Minority Rights Group
379 Brixton Road
London SW9
Tel: 0171 978 9498

*National Association of
Community Relations Councils*
8–16 Coronet Street
London N1 6HD
Tel: 0171 739 6658

*National Black Community Care
Forum*
High Holborn House
49–51 Bedford Row
London WC1V 6DJ
Tel: 0171 430 0811

*National Health Service Ethnic
Health Unit*
7 Belmont Grove
Leeds LS2 9NP
Tel: 0113 246 7336

Overseas Doctors Association
28–32 Princess Street
Manchester M1 4LB
Tel: 0161 236 5594

The Refugee Council
3 Bondway
London SW8 1SJ
Tel: 0171 582 6922

SHARE
The King's Fund Centre
11–13 Cavendish Square
London W1M 0AN
Tel: 0171 307 2686

Sia, Black Development Agency
High Holborn House
49–51 Bedford Row
London WC1V 6DJ
Tel: 0171 430 0811

Sickle Cell Society
54 Station Road
Harlesden
London NW10 4UA
Tel: 0181 961 7795

*Standing Conference of
West Indian Organisations in
Great Britain*
5 Westminster Bridge Road
London SE1 7XW
Tel: 0171 928 7861

*Thalassaemia Society,
United Kingdom*
107 Nightingale Lane
London N8 7QV
Tel: 0181 348 0437

*United Kingdom Immigrants
Advisory Service (UKIAS)*
190 Great Dover Street
London SE1 4YB
Tel: 0171 357 6917

Asians

Anil Bhalla
Asian Resource Centre
101 Villa Road
Handsworth
Birmingham B19 1NH
Tel: 0121 5230580

Jahinder Bhuhi
Mental Health Development Worker
Gusford Asian Group
East Street
Coventry CV1 5LS
Tel: 01203 555497

Bradford Community Health Trust
Zeenat Hussain, Co-ordinator
Ethnic Minority Development
Service
Leeds Road Hospital
Maudsley Street
Bradford BD3 9LH
Tel: 01274 363450

Bradford Health Commission
Selina Ullah, Development Manager
New Mill
Victoria Road
Saltaire, Near Shipley
Bradford BD18 3LB
Tel: 01274 366006
Fax: 01274 366060

Razia Shamin
Ethnic Action Worker
Age Concern
Metro Rochdale
38 Long Street
Manchester M24 3UQ
Tel: 0161 6532157

*Roshni Asian Women's Resource
Centre*
Abda Sadiq, Co-ordinator
444 London Road
Sheffield S2 4HP
Tel: 0114 2508898

Bosnians

Bosnia Project
Refugee Council
3/9 Bondway
London SW8 1SJ
Tel: 0171 582 6922

Xenia Wilding
Bosnia Herzegovina Advice Centre
10 Rosslyn Court
Ornan Road
London NW3 4PU
Tel: 0171 435 4180

Latin Americans

Latin American Bureau
1 Amwell Street
London EC1R 1EL
Tel: 0171 278 2829

Latin America Section
Refugee Council
3/9 Bondway
London SW8 1SJ
Tel: 0171 582 6922

Index

Under each *religion*, in the text, will be found a standard list of headings; use these for further details.